Curbside Consultation
of the Spine

49 Clinical Questions

CURBSIDE CONSULTATION IN ORTHOPEDICS
SERIES

SERIES EDITOR, BERNARD R. BACH, JR., MD

Curbside Consultation
of the Spine

49 Clinical Questions

Kern Singh, MD

Assistant Professor, Division of Spine Surgery
Department of Orthopaedic Surgery
Rush University Medical Center
Midwest Orthopaedic at Rush
Chicago, IL

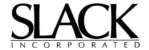

SLACK
INCORPORATED

Delivering the best in health care information and education worldwide

www.slackbooks.com

ISBN: 978-1-55642-823-4

The procedures and practices described in this book should be implemented in a manner consistent with the professional standards set for the circumstances that apply in each specific situation. Every effort has been made to confirm the accuracy of the information presented and to correctly relate generally accepted practices. The authors, editor, and publisher cannot accept responsibility for errors or exclusions or for the outcome of the material presented herein. There is no expressed or implied warranty of this book or information imparted by it. Care has been taken to ensure that drug selection and dosages are in accordance with currently accepted/recommended practice. Due to continuing research, changes in government policy and regulations, and various effects of drug reactions and interactions, it is recommended that the reader carefully review all materials and literature provided for each drug, especially those that are new or not frequently used. Any review or mention of specific companies or products is not intended as an endorsement by the author or publisher.

SLACK Incorporated uses a review process to evaluate submitted material. Prior to publication, educators or clinicians provide important feedback on the content that we publish. We welcome feedback on this work.

Published by: SLACK Incorporated
                   6900 Grove Road
                   Thorofare, NJ 08086 USA
                   Telephone: 856-848-1000
                   Fax: 856-848-6091
                   www.slackbooks.com

Contact SLACK Incorporated for more information about other books in this field or about the availability of our books from distributors outside the United States.

Curbside consultation of the spine : 49 clinical questions / [edited by] Kern Singh.
     p. ; cm. -- (Curbside consultation in orthopedics)
  Includes bibliographical references and index.
  ISBN 978-1-55642-823-4
  1. Spine--Surgery--Miscellanea. I. Singh, Kern. II. Series.
  [DNLM: 1. Spine--surgery. 2. Spinal Diseases--surgery. WE 725 C975 2008]
  RD768.C87 2008
  617.5'6059--dc22
                                      2008010381

Printed in the United States of America.

Last digit is print number: 10   9   8   7   6   5   4   3   2   1

Dedication

This book is dedicated to my mother,
whose never-ending sacrifices from the past
have given me my immeasurable successes of today.

Contents

Acknowledgments

I would like to thank all the contributing authors for their outstanding support. This book reflects what I believe to be a collection of the future leaders in spine surgery. It was an honor to be able to assemble an all-star team of young spine surgeons who also happen to be close friends and colleagues. I would also like to thank the staff at SLACK Incorporated, and in particular Carrie Kotlar, for helping to put together this outstanding text. Never did I think putting together a book would be so easy... clearly it was due to the amazing help from all the contributors at SLACK! Lastly, I would like to thank Bernie Bach, MD. He was a mentor when I was a resident and is a true friend and colleague now that we are partners. Without him I would not have had this opportunity to put together this textbook.

Kern Singh, MD

About the Editor

Kern Singh, MD graduated from the Pennsylvania State University in 1995, Jefferson Medical College in 1999, and completed his Orthopaedic Surgery residency at Rush University Medical Center (1999 to 2004). He completed a Spine Surgery fellowship at Emory University in 2005 before returning to join the staff of the Department of Orthopedics, Section of Spine Surgery, at Rush University Medical Center as an assistant professor. Dr. Singh currently serves as an editor for the *Journal of American Academy of Orthopedic Surgery, American Journal of Orthopedics*, and the *Journal of Contemporary Spine Surgery*. He has co-authored multiple technique and review articles, book chapters, and peer-reviewed manuscripts in the field of spine surgery. Additionally, he has served as a faculty member for both national and international courses in Spine Surgery.

Contributing Authors

Shay Bess, MD
San Diego Center for Spinal Disorders
La Jolla, CA

Rick A. Davis, MD
Assistant Professor of Orthopedic Surgery
Adult Spine Surgery
Director, Minimally Invasive Orthopedic
    Spine Center
Vanderbilt University Medical Center
Nashville, TN

Brian Kwon, MD
Clinical Instructor
Department Orthopedic Surgery
Tufts University School of Medicine
New England Baptist Hospital
Boston, MA

Joon Y. Lee, MD
Assistant Professor
Orthopaedic and Neurological Surgery
University of Pittsburgh Medical Center
Pittsburgh, PA

Yu-Po Lee, MD
UCSD Dept. of Orthopaedic Surgery
San Diego, CA

Ahmad Nassr, MD
Senior Associate Consultant
Department of Orthopedic Surgery
Instructor of Orthopedic Surgery
Mayo Clinic College of Medicine
Rochester, MN

Alpesh A. Patel, MD
Assistant Professor
Department of Orthopaedic Surgery
Department of Neurosurgery
University of Utah School of Medicine
Salt Lake City, UT

Joseph D. Smucker, MD
Assistant Professor
The University of Iowa
Dept. of Orthopaedics and Rehabilitation
Iowa City, IA

Preface

It is my firm belief that of all the disciplines in medicine, the field of spine surgery has seen the most rapid growth and evolution in the last ten years. While still in its infancy, spine surgery has advanced significantly from the days of body casts and traction to image guidance and percutaneous instrumentation. Ironically, the gargantuan advancement in spinal technology has clearly outpaced our ability to answer some of the most fundamental clinical scenarios in spine. The management of simple issues such as back and neck pain, disc herniations, and spinal cord compression vary from surgeon and institution. Current spinal textbooks are often inundated with extensive tomes of anatomic information and historical references that offer the reader very little practical information regarding the management of common clinical scenarios. As such, I believe that this text is directed at answering those very situations that are often left unaddressed in the "gold-standard" textbooks of spinal surgery. What better way to address current clinical dilemmas then to ask the "young stars" in spine surgery their opinions? Readers will find a refreshingly succinct yet poignant text that provides answers to those very questions that spinal surgeons encounter on a daily basis. It is my hope that this textbook provides readers with "curbside answers" from the leading young authorities in the field of spine surgery.

Kern Singh, MD

Foreword

Dear Reader,

It is the nature of medical progress that increasing insight into a given field reveals complexity and begets sub-specialization. Thus, one's initial exposure to the field of spinal disorders, whether as a medical student or resident in orthopedic surgery or neurosurgery, can be rather intimidating. Dr. Singh and colleagues have compiled a series of answers to common and relevant questions in the evaluation and treatment of spinal disease. Practical aspects of diagnosis and management are addressed in pertinent areas ranging from the outpatient setting to the operating room, from pediatric to aged patients, and from the mundane manifestations of disc degeneration to more uncommon and complex issues such as spinal tumors and infections.

The nature of this primer is to help orient the novice in the field to the bigger picture. It provides an intellectual compass to help guide one through early experiences in the field. Pertinent references follow each chapter, which invite more in-depth reading on a given topic. With the understanding that further reading is essential to meaningful learning in this field, as in any other, Dr. Singh and colleagues are to be commended for providing thumbnail sketches of common clinical settings to assist young physicians in the care of the spine.

Sincerely,
John G. Heller, MD
Professor of Orthopaedic Surgery
The Emory Clinic
Emory University
Atlanta, GA

SECTION I

ANATOMY

1

HOW DO I KNOW INTRAOPERATIVELY THAT I HAVE DONE A THOROUGH LUMBAR DECOMPRESSION?

Rick A. Davis, MD

Lumbar spinal stenosis is defined as a narrowing of the spinal canal that produces compression of the neural elements. The lumbar canal can be divided into three zones: the central, lateral recess, and the pedicle/neuroforamen.[1] Central spinal stenosis commonly occurs at the disc level as a result of facet joint overgrowth.[1] Specifically, the inferior articular process of the cephalad vertebrae is located dorsal and medial, and contributes to the lateral osseous wall of the central spinal canal.[1] The formation of osteophytes on this articular process results in focal narrowing of the central spinal canal.[1] The lateral recess zone is the area between the lateral border of the dural sac along the median and a longitudinal line connecting the medial walls of the pedicles laterally.[1] Lateral recess stenosis affects the traversing spinal nerve root at the disc level and at the superior aspect of the pedicle. In contrast, the superior articular process of the caudal vertebrae is located lateral and ventral.[1] Osteophytic enlargement of this process in response to facet degeneration results in narrowing of the lateral recess and neural foramen.[1]

When considering surgery, it is beneficial to identify all areas of stenosis that require decompression. A standard wide decompressive laminectomy involves removal of the lamina and ligamentum flavum from the lateral border of one lateral recess to that of the other at all involved spinal levels.[1] I like to use the medial wall of the pedicle to identify the lateral extent of my central and lateral recess decompression. This is a reliable method to ensure adequate decompression. In addition, it maintains an appropriate amount of the pars interarticularis, thereby preventing the possibility of an iatrogenic pars fracture (Figure 1-1). It is important to probe each foramen (Figure 1-2) and consider a foramen decompressed when you can move a ball-point probe freely in all four directions. I always leave at least 1 cm of the pars and at least 50% of each facet joint if I am not going to fuse that level. Limited intraoperative myelography combined with intraoperative CT scanning might prove to be the most reliable tool to use in the future.

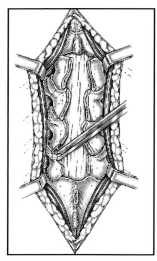

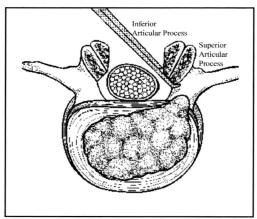

Figure 1-2. A kerrison rongeur is used to undercut the superior orticular process, ensuring that the neuroforamen is decompressed..

Figure 1-1. A central decompression has been accomplished and a kerrison rongeur is being used to perform a resection of the lateral recess.

Reference

1. Spivak JM. Current concepts review: degenerative lumbar spinal stenosis. *JBJS*. 1998;80-A(7):1053-1066.

WHEN PERFORMING A LUMBAR MICRODISCECTOMY, IS IT BETTER TO PERFORM ONLY A FRAGMENTECTOMY OR SHOULD I PERFORM AN ANNULOTOMY AND BE MORE AGGRESSIVE ABOUT THE DISC REMOVAL?

Rick A. Davis, MD

Unsuccessful surgical treatment, including the occurrence of a disc reherniation following lumbar discectomy, is a significant problem in the modern treatment of herniated nucleus pulposus. Previous studies have shown that the recurrence of radiculopathy and reherniation rates following discectomy can be as high as 33%. Historically, discectomy has been performed via a large annulotomy with the removal of as much loose disc material as possible to decrease the likelihood of reherniation. I prefer to use a less invasive method termed a fragmentectomy or a limited discectomy (Figure 2-1). This method involves the removal of only extruded fragments, leaving the internal nuclear architecture intact. Intraoperatively, I also find the annulotomy defect and probe it with a nerve hook and penfield elevator to determine if there are any residual fragments that may be gently released. At no point do I place a pituitary rongeur or curette into the disc space, because I feel this only accelerates the damage to the internal structure of the disc.

I inform my patients that with this limited approach discectomy there is an increased risk of reherniation. For me, the benefits of preserving as much intervertebral disc as possible clearly outweigh the possibility of a recurrent disc herniation. I instruct all patients with large annular defects (>6 mm) to avoid strenuous activity for the first 6 weeks after the operation. Large annular defects are the single greatest risk factor for recurrent disc herniation, and as such, I am much more protective of these patients.

Despite a higher reherniation rate, patients in the limited discectomy group have significantly better visual analog scale (VAS) (back) and Oswestry scores at 6 and 12 months than patients in the sub-total discectomy group (with no difference at 2 years) and also

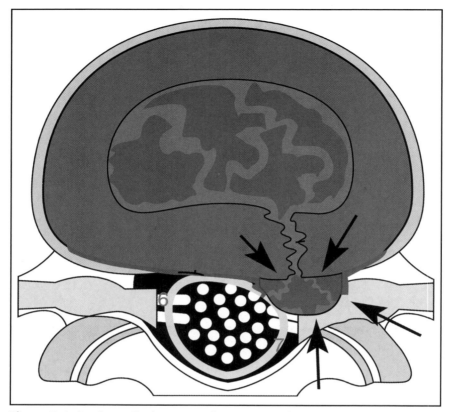

Figure 2-1. A schematic demonstrating a posterolateral disc herniation with extravasation of the nuclear contents causing abutment of the spinal nerve root.

require less pain medication after surgery. Carragee et al[1] also demonstrated that the limited discectomy group experienced a significantly shorter convalescent period and continued to work in heavier occupation categories with fewer restrictions. It should be noted that although the majority of patients in both groups (limited discectomy versus subtotal discectomy) were ultimately satisfied with outcomes, at all follow-up points the satisfaction level with outcomes was statistically better in the limited discectomy group.

Reference

1. Carragee EJ, Spinnickie AO, Alamin TF, Paragioudakis S. A prospective controlled study of limited versus subtotal posterior diskectomy: Short-term outcomes in patients with hernaited lumbar invertebral discs and large posterior anular defects. *Spine.* 2006;31(6):653-657.

I AM GOING TO PERFORM AN ANTERIOR THORACIC SPINAL RELEASE. ARE THERE ANY INTRAOPERATIVE PRECAUTIONS I CAN TAKE TO MINIMIZE THE RISK OF SPINAL CORD INFARCTION?

Rick A. Davis, MD

Since the 1960s, surgeons have been anxious about the potential for paraplegia that may result from litigation of the segmental vessels on the lateral side of the vertebral bodies when performing anterior spine surgery. The ligation of these segmental vessels has been reported to result in spinal cord ischemia because of the lack of collateral circulation in some patients[1] (Figure 3-1). Ischemic damage usually occurs secondary to occlusion of the anterior spinal artery or radicular arteries.[2] In a retrospective review of 1197 consecutive anterior operative procedures, Winter et al[1] revealed no evidence of paraplegia related to segmental vessel ligation. Others have reported a paraplegia rate of 0.51% to 0.65% and an incomplete rate between 0.41% and 1.25%.[2] Winter et al attributed these results to several factors[1]:

1. Never use hypotensive anesthesia because this may contribute to lower spinal cord blood flow from the collateral circulation.

2. Divide the segmental vessels at the midportion of the vertebral body and never close to the neuroforamen, where important collateral vessels can exist.

3. Always approach scoliosis from the convexity of the curve. Arteries on the convexity are typically smaller than on the concavity, suggesting that there is less blood flow on this side of the deformity.

4. Never ligate vessels on both sides at the same level.

Although some authors have suggested using spinal cord monitoring, I have found no utility to the temporary clamping of vessels with somatosensory-evoked potential moni-

Figure 3-1. A magnetic resonance angiogram demonstrating the segmental blood supply of the thoracic spine..

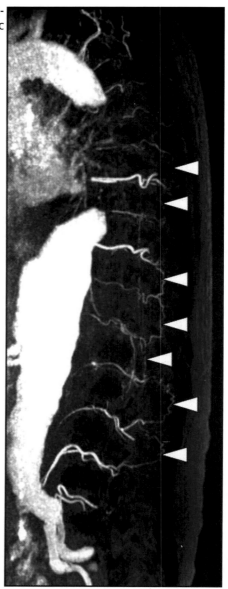

toring.[1,2] Spinal cord injury after deformity surgery may also result from a mechanical injury, ie misplaced instrumentation, misplaced bone graft, and postoperative hematoma. Surgeons should be cognizant of these factors because they may be the source of the signal change. Other risks factors for spinal cord injury include short-curve kyphosis correction versus long-curve kyphosis, large correctional angles, congenital malformations, hypovascularity of the spinal cord in the midthoracic region, coagulopathy, and pre-existing neurologic deficits.[2] Although spinal cord ischemia is a real phenomenon, several protective measures can be taken to reduce the likelihood of disastrous neurological compromise.

References

1. Winter RB, Lonstein JE, Denis F, Leonard A, Garamella J. Paraplegia resulting from vessel ligation. *Spine.* 1996;12(10):1232-1233.
2. Baron EM. Medical complications of surgical treatment of adult spinal deformity and how to avoid them. *Spine.* 2006;31(19):106-118.

SECTION II

DIAGNOSTIC IMAGING

I HAVE A PATIENT WITH DEGENERATIVE DISC DISEASE AT L5-S1 THAT IS CLINICALLY SYMPTOMATIC. WHAT IS A DISCOGRAM AND WHEN SHOULD I ORDER ONE?

Rick A. Davis, MD

After an extended course of conservative treatment, discography can be used in an attempt to identify the disc as the pain generator. Based on pressure, morphology, and pain concordance, discography is used to determine if dark discs are painful and surrounding discs are painless (Figure 4-1).

The Executive Committee of the North American Spine Society issued its indications for discography in a recent position statement[1]:

1. Unremitting spinal pain, with or without extremity pain, of greater than 4 months in duration, not responsive to any standard method of conservative treatment

2. Persistent disc-related pain, suspected when other evaluation modalities are equivocal

3. Persistent pain in the postoperative period as a result of suspected intervertebral disk degeneration, recurrent herniation, or pseudarthrosis

4. Disc space evaluation in a spine segment considered for fusion to determine whether it is a pain generator

5. Determination of primary symptom-producing level or levels when chemonucleolysis or other intradiscal procedures are being contemplated

Discography involves introducing a needle into the nucleus pulpous of the target disc and distending the disc from the inside with an injection of contrast medium to try to reproduce pain that is believed to be discal in eitology.[1] This contrast medium is then used to outline the disc's morphology. There are the 2 distinct phases of discography:

Figure 4-1. Fluoroscopic discogram evaluating a normal discogram at L2-3, L3-4, and L4-5 with an abnormal posterial leak at L5-S1.

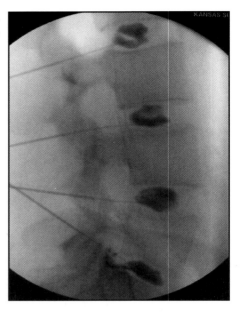

disc stimulation and internal morphology evaluation. Disc stimulation denotes that during the pressurization of the disc, several variables are recorded: the patient's pain response (VAS score), pressure required to simulate pain, and the concordance of the pain. Concordant pain is pain that is similar in nature to what the patient experiences every day. The opening pressures for the injections are valuable to use in correlation with the pain response.

A computed tomography (CT) scan is then performed to check the position of the dye used in the discogram and to evaluate the morphology of the disc. The disc morphology is then graded based on the amount of leakage or degeneration. False positives can occur with annulus and endplate injections. It is important to not oversedate the patient during the discogram because the patient needs to be able to verbalize his or her pain response. A painful disc leaks from the center either posteriorly toward the canal or peripherally in the annulus. If more volume is required, a tear may be indicated, because the normal volume of a lumbar disc is between 0.5 to 1.5 cc.

There are several criteria for establishing a positive discogram: (1) abnormal morphology including posterior annular disruption, (2) pain concordant to the patient's usual pain, (3) pain limited to 1 or 2 disk levels, and (4) a negative control.

Discography is evolving to play a critical role in the evaluation of axial low back pain, especially in regards to surgical decision making.[1] Discography remains the only test that seeks to provoke a pain response in selected patients with recalcitrant back pain. It should be noted however, that discography remains a second-line diagnostic modality.

Reference

1. Guyer RD, Ohnmeiss DD. Lumbar discography: position statement from the North American Spine Society Diagnostic and Therapeutic Committee. *Spine.* 1995;20:2048-2059.

I HAVE A 34-YEAR-OLD MALE WITH RECURRENT LEG PAIN 4 WEEKS AFTER A DISCECTOMY. WHAT IMAGING STUDY SHOULD I ORDER?

Rick A. Davis, MD

Lumbar discectomy in a patient with severe intractable sciatica can be one of the most successful surgeries. However, a number of patients do not improve, rapidly relapse, have recurrent herniations, or develop disabling axial symptoms. Depending on the series reviewed, up to 20% to 40% of discectomies done for herniated lumbar intervertebral discs result in serious postoperative difficulties. Carragee et al analyzed 250 patients; their analysis indicated that magnetic resonance imaging (MRI) findings of fragment type, herniation size, and shape were the most consistent predictors of clinical results.[1] They empirically grouped their experience into four categories:

1. Extruded fragments with minimal annular defects

2. Extruded fragments with large annular defects

3. Contained disc herniations

4. Contained annular prolaspe without clear fragments

The authors found that group 2 accounted for all of the multiple disc reherniations and concluded that the primary predictor of outcome was disc herniation size and the remaining competency of the annulus fibrosus.

Distinction between scar and disc has been attempted with myelography, computed tomography, discography, and magenetic resonance imaging (MRI). The clinical significance of MRI findings in relation to symptoms and clinical signs can be confusing in low back pain patients with or without sciatica. Contrast medium (gadolinium) is routinely used in MRI after disc operations (in hopes of delineating epidural fibrosis and recurrent

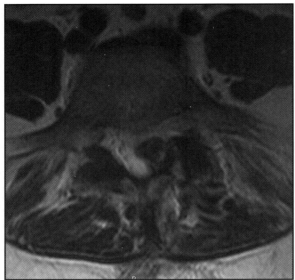

Figure 5-1. A 51-year-old female with a large left sided L4-5 Recurrent HNP (extruded disc fragment) two weeks after surgery.

disc herniation). In patients with low back pain, rim enhancement around disc herniations is thought to represent a combination of neovascularized granulation tissue and epidural venous plexus. It is generally accepted that patients who undergo operations for recurrent disc herniation tend to make progress, whereas those in whom only epidural fibrosis is found at surgery tend to show little improvement.[2]

It has become routine practice at many institutions to perform contrast-enhanced examinations (using gadolinium) whenever studying postoperative patients with recurrent low back pain and/or radiculopathy. These recommendations may have evolved because limitations in technology may no longer apply (ie, prolonged imaging times for T2-weighted imaging on low-field-strength scanners).

References

1. Carragee EJ, Han mY, Suen PW, Kim D. Clinical outcomes after lumbar discectomy for sciatica: The effects of fragment type and annular competence. *American Journal of Bone and Joint Surgery.* 2003;85-A(1):102-108.
2. Autio RA. Gadolinium diethylenetriaminepentaacetic acid enhancement in magnetic resonance imaging in relation to symptoms and signs among sciatic patients. *Spine.* 2002;27(13):1433-1437.

I HAVE A PATIENT WITH A SMALL DISK HERNIATION BUT HE CONTINUES TO COMPLAIN OF RIGHT LOWER EXTREMITY RADICULOPATHY. IS THERE AN IMAGING STUDY OR TEST I CAN ORDER TO HELP ME CONFIRM MY DIAGNOSIS?

Rick A. Davis, MD

It is important to perform a thorough history and physical examination because people who complain of leg pain may have other sources of pathology. Common etiologies of leg pain may include hip and knee arthritis, greater trochanter bursitis, pseudo-radicular pain from sacroiliitis, and vascular claudication.

There are several tests that can be performed to help clear up a confusing situation. A discogram can be used if a patient complains of only back pain and has an MRI scan that is difficult to interpret.[1] In this same situation, if the patient complains of leg pain, a CT myelogram may provide more detailed information regarding the patency of the neuroforamen. An electromyogram (EMG) can used to help identify a peripheral neuropathy (ie, diabetes) versus a true lumbar radiculopathy. The EMG may be subjective because the results depend on the experience of the technician, and in my practice it very rarely notes a true radiculopathy. Polyradiculopathy, often with bilateral involvement of multiple levels, is a typical pattern in symptomatic stenotic patients.[2] The evaluation of somatosensory-evoked potentials both before and after exercise may help to determine which nerve roots are most involved in central spinal canal stenosis at the lumbar level in question.

If all these tests still do not identify the pathology, then I perform a transforaminal epidural steroid injection (TFESI) or a selective nerve root block. I do these injections myself because I can gather useful information. A TFESI helps to provide immediate pain relief to the patient and can provide a long-term therapeutic benefit. Furthermore, during the injection, the patient's pain can be reproduced when the contrast medium or steroid is injected. This information is invaluable in confirming if the nerve root is the etiology of the patient's lower extremity pain. If the TFESI reproduces the patient's pain during the injection of the contrast medium and if the anesthetic relieves the patient's symptoms, I feel extremely confident in diagnosing the small disc herniation as the source of the radiculopathy.

References

1. Whitaker C, Hochschuler S. *Pocket Spine.* St Louis, MO: Quality Medical Publishers; 2006.
2. Spivak JM. Degenerative lumbar spinal stenosis. *J Bone Joint Surg Am.* 1998;80(7):1053-1066.

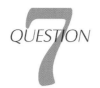

I Have a 34-Year-Old Female With a Discogram Positive L5-S1 Degenerative Disc Who Wants to Avoid Surgery at All Costs. Is Intradiscal Electrothermal Therapy a Reasonable Alternative?

Rick A. Davis, MD

There is no place for intradiscal electrothermal therapy (IDET) in my practice. The technology has limited benefit and very little clinical evidence to support its use in patients. In IDET, a coil is placed into the disc space (Figure 7-1). The coil temperature is then increased, theoretically destroying the nociceptive fibers found in the outer annulus. Theoretically, the IDET also causes a remodeling of the collagen fibers that help reduce painful motion. Basic scientific studies do not support the theory behind the IDET, and clinical results are just as mixed. Most studies do not show improvement over the natural history; this technique is best performed on young, large discs; and the results are only 50/50 at best.[1]

The Saal brothers were instrumental in the development of IDET and have been the only physicians to report and publish success with this technology. Saal et al found that 80% of patients reported a reduction of 2 points in the visual analog pain scale and 72% discontinued pain medication.[2] Karasek and Bogduk found 60% benefited 1 year following treatment and 23% reported improvement in VAS pain scores as compared to physical therapy alone.[3]

Freeman et al performed a randomized, double-blind controlled efficacy study: IDET vs placebo. The control group had an inactive probe inserted into the intervertebral disc, whereas the experimental group was treated with an active IDET probe.[4] The physician and patient were blinded to the treatment. All patients completed a standardized reha-

Figure 7-1. A fluoroscope image demonstrating an IDET coil inserted into the L4-5 disc space.

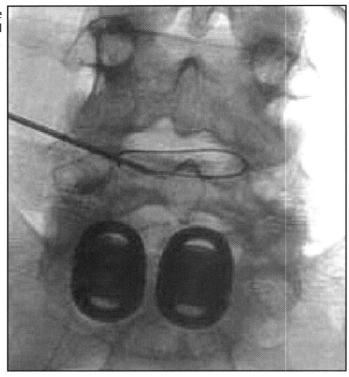

bilitation program. At the 6-month follow-up, 55 of 57 patients had completed the study. No improvement was noted in the SF-36, Zung Depression Index (ZDI), or the Modified Somatic Perceptions Questionnaire (MSPQ). Additionally, no significant improvement in either treatment group was noted when comparing pre- to post-treatment scores.[4] In my opinion, this study confirms that there is no significant benefit from IDET over placebo.

References

1. Herkowitz H. *Surgical Options for "Discogenic" Low Back Pain.* AAOS Instructional Course, 2002.
2. Saal JS, Saal JA. Management of chronic discogenic low back pain with a thermal intradiscal catheter: a preliminary report. *Spine.* 2000:25(3):382-388.
3. Karasek M, Bogduk N. Twelve-month follow-up of a control trial of intradiscal thermal anuloplasty for back pain due to internal disc disruption. *Spine.* 2000:25(20):2601-2607.
4. Freeman BJC, Fraser RD, Christopher MJ, et al. A randomized, double-blind, controlled trial: intradiscal electrothermal therapy versus placebo for the treatment of chronic discogenic low back pain. *Spine.* 2005;30:2369-2377.

I HAVE PATIENTS WITH SPINAL STENOSIS AND OTHERS WITH FORAMINAL STENOSIS AND FACET DEGENERATION. WHAT TYPES OF ANESTHETIC INJECTIONS ARE AVAILABLE AND WHEN SHOULD I ORDER THEM?

Rick A. Davis, MD

I think you have to first separate out the cause of the leg and back pain. Stenosis can cause neurogenic claudication and referred pain into the lower extremities with concomitant back pain. Musculoskeletal pathology, facet arthropathy, and degenerative disc disease all may be possible etiologies of back pain as well.

Regardless of the injection performed, no procedure should be done without fluoroscopic guidance because of the associated high failure rate.[1] The literature has conflicting reports concerning the value of interlaminar epidural steroid injections. It is questionable whether traditional epidural injections (both caudal and interlaminar types) deliver an adequate concentration of anesthetic and corticosteroid to the neural elements.[1] In a prospective, randomized, double-blinded study, Cuckler et al found no statistically significant difference with interlaminar injections as compared to placebo injections.[2]

I believe a more effective type of injection is a transforaminal epidural steroid (TFESI) or selective nerve root block. Despite the fact that selective nerve root injections have been described for years, few studies regarding their efficacy have been completed until recently. Riew et al[3] looked at 55 patients with a diagnosis of stenosis or disc herniation causing lumbar radicular pain. All patients who were treated with a selective nerve root block delayed the need for a surgical decompression for as long as 28 months.[3] The authors concluded that patients who have lumbar radicular pain at 1 or 2 levels should be considered for treatment with nerve root blocks of corticosteroids prior to being considered for operative treatment. Not only do a TFESI and a nerve root block reduce the patient's pain, but also they provide insight into the correct diagnosis.

There are more than 4 four possible mechanisms of action to explain the high efficacy of TFESIs[1] (Figure 8-1):

Figure 8-1. A fluoroscopic image of a typical cervical TFESI.

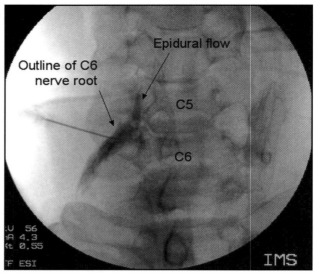

1. Precise delivery of steroid and xylocaine solution to the ventral aspect of the lumbar nerve root sleeve and the dorsal aspect of the disc herniation

2. Nerve-membrane–stabilizing properties of both the steroid and xylocaine

3. A "washout" effect of the solution that decreases the regional levels of inflammatory mediators

4. Potent anti-inflammatory properties of the corticosteroid

Facet dysfunction or pain can present in 3% of patients with failed back surgery[4] and in 15 to 40% of patients with chronic low back pain.[5] The literature has noted variable correlation among history, physical exam, CT, and radiographs.[4] Facet injections, medial branch blocks, and rhizotomies have been used for the diagnosis and treatment of low back pain.[4-7] Unfortunately the literature is sparse and conflicting at best. As such, I do not routinely prescribe facet injections because of the uncertainty in regards to their treatment efficacy.[7]

References

1. Vad VB, Bhat AL, Lutz GE, et al. Transforaminal epidural steroid injections in lumbosacral radiculopathy: a prospective randomized study. *Spine.* 2007;27(1):11-16.
2. Cuckler JM, Bernini PA, Wiesel S, et al. The use of epidural steroids in the treatment of lumbar radicular pain: a prospective, randomized, double-blind study. *J Bone Joint Surg Am.* 1985;67(1):63-66.
3. Riew, DK. The effect of nerve-root injections on the need for operative treatment of lumbar radicular pain. *J Bone Joint Surg Am.* 2000;82:11-17.
4. Schwarzer AC, Aprill CN, Derby R, et al. Clinical features of patients with pain stemming from the lumbar zygapophyseal joints: is the lumbar facet syndrome a clinical entity? *Spine.* 1994;19(10):1132-1137.
5. Dreyfuss P, Michaelsen M, Pauza K, et al. The value of medical history and physical examination in diagnosing sacroiliac joint pain. *Spine.* 1996;21(22):2594-2602.
6. Schofferman J. A prospective randomized comparison of 270° fusions to 360° fusions (circumferential fusions). *Spine.* 2001;26(10):E207-212.
7. Schwarzer AC, Aprill CN, Bogduk N. The sacroiliac joint in chronic low back pain. *Spine.* 1995;20:31-37.

SECTION III

SURGICAL APPROACH

I Have a Lot of Patients With L5-S1 Degenerative Disc Disease. What Surgical Options Do I Have for Accessing the Anterior L5-S1 Interspace?

Joseph D. Smucker, MD

L5-S1 degenerative disc disease is a common pathologic entity, and many surgical interventions have been entertained for the treatment of this condition. It has been my experience that indications are the most important factor in determining surgical success in the treatment of this condition.

Access to the L5-S1 interspace can be challenging because of the presence of the pelvis and abdominal vasculature. The iliac crests almost always interfere with a direct lateral approach. Although it is possible to perform a transforaminal lumbar interbody fusion (TLIF) procedure at this interspace, it is my personal experience that the exposure is typically limited and more difficult to accomplish. A posterior lumbar interbody fusion (PLIF) may be accomplished at the L5-S1 interval as a way to posteriorally access the intervertebral disc. Challenges with the PLIF at this level include excessive retraction of the neural elements. A new procedure, the AxiaLIF, makes use of a reverse Herbert screw technique to create an L5-S1 fusion via a percutaneous approach. Disc removal, a key component of any interbody fusion procedure, is incomplete in all procedures except anterior lumbar interbody fusion (ALIF). Successful fusion with any of these techniques demands enough disc removal to allow for sufficient bony growth from endplate to endplate.

ALIF is my preferred technique for accessing the L5-S1 intervertebral level. An anterior approach may be accomplished in several different ways and is often specific to the institution and the surgeon. Some institutions rely heavily on approach surgeons, general or vascular surgeons, who can assist with access to this disc space. Some surgeons pre-

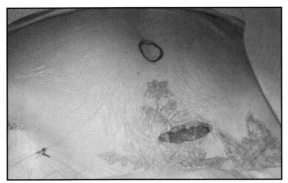

Figure 9-1. A typical incision made for a retroperitoneal approach to the L5-S1 disc space.

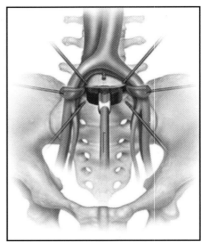

Figure 9-2. A schematic demostrating retraction of the external iliac vein with insertion of an ALIF cage.

fer to accomplish this approach on their own, and as such the approach is made much easier with good surgical assistance and the absence of prior abdominal or pelvic surgery and/or radiation. Finally, an ALIF may also be performed via a laparoscopic approach. This has been well described, although the relative advantages of this approach over the standard open approach have been debated, and the increase in results are marginal at best.[1]

It is important to understand the preoperative vascular anatomy of those patients you choose to access via an anterior route.[2] The iliac artery and vein bifurcate in this region. The bifurcation typically occurs at or just above the L5-S1 interspace (Figures 9-1 and 9-2). In many cases this presents an ideal access for a direct anterior approach after a retroperitoneal or transperitoneal dissection has been accomplished. The case is certainly made more challenging if the bifurcation occurs below the L5-S1 interval because appropriate mobilization of the vasculature may be difficult.

References

1. Rodriguez HE, Connolly MM, Dracopoulos H, et al. Anterior access to the lumbar spine: laparoscopic versus open. *Am Surg.* 2002;68:978-982.
2. Vraney RT, Phillips FM, Wetzel FT, et al. Peridiscal vascular anatomy of the lower lumbar spine: an endoscopic perspective. *Spine.* 1999;24:2183-2187.

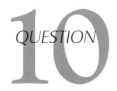

10

I Have a Patient With Discogenic Pain and a Symptomatic L3-4 Intervertebral Disc. What Are My Options?

Joseph D. Smucker, MD

At the L3-4 intervertebral level, common anterior challenges include the vasculature of the aorta and vena cava. Mobilization of the surrounding vasculature at these levels is the key to adequate anterior exposure.[1] Surgeons discuss with males of child-bearing age that a disruption to the sympathetic plexus may result in retrograde ejaculation in a minority of patients.

Although anterior lumbar interbody fusion (ALIF) remains the gold standard for complete disc resection, transforaminal lumbar interbody fusion (TLIF) is an excellent alternative that avoids the challenges of an anterior dissection.[2] TLIF typically involves the complete resection of a unilateral lumbar facet and transforaminal discectomy. At the L3-4 interspace, identification and mobilization of the exiting nerve root is appropriate prior to the discectomy. A TLIF typically allows for a more aggressive discectomy than a PLIF, as well as possible placement of a larger interbody implant with minimal neural retraction.

Posterior lumbar interbody fusion (PLIF) is a second posteriorly based approach to the L3-4 intervertebral disc that has been used by surgeons for many years.[3] A PLIF involves moderate resection of the medial portion of the facets at the L3-4 interspace. Careful identification and exposure of the thecal sac and neural elements are critical portions of this procedure. PLIF is often accomplished through annulotomies to the right and left side of the dural sac. To accomplish a thorough discectomy via this technique, it is often necessary to retract the neural elements more aggressively than is needed in a routine discectomy. The surgeon must be very cautious not to retract entrapped neural elements or to continuously retract elements in an aggressive manner.

Extreme lateral interbody fusion (XLIF) is a procedure developed to address the challenges of the three previously mentioned interbody fusion techniques.[4] With the patient

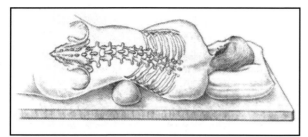

Figure 10-1. Patient position for an XLIF with a bump underneath the affected level..

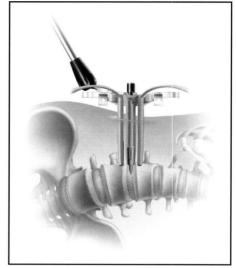

Figure 10-2. Minimally invasive retractor system docked into the disc space.

in the direct lateral position, a minimally invasive retroperitoneal approach is accomplished with the use of a modified retractor system and fluoroscopic localization of the intervertebral disc from the lateral view (Figures 10-1 and 10-2).

XLIF involves a direct lateral approach to the L3-4 intervertebral disc via a trans-psoas approach. Continuous electromyography (EMG) monitoring is typically used to identify the presence of neural elements during the approach. XLIF carries the unique distinction of preserving both the anterior and posterior longitudinal ligaments of the spine. This is an attractive biomechanical advantage in that interbody implants may be less likely to be displaced. XLIF allows for a maximal discectomy that is similar to an ALIF. XLIF is unable to access the L5-S1 disc space because of the proximity of the pelvis and ilium. XLIF is best utilized for direct approaches to the upper and middle lumbar intervertebral segments.

References

1. Vraney RT, Phillips FM, Wetzel FT, et al. Peridiscal vascular anatomy of the lower lumbar spine: an endoscopic perspective. *Spine.* 1999;24:2183-2187.
2. Hackenberg L, Halm H, Bullmann V, et al. Transforaminal lumbar interbody fusion: a safe technique with satisfactory three to five year results. *Eur Spine J.* 2005;14:551-558.
3. Brislin B, Vaccaro AR. Advances in posterior lumbar interbody fusion. *Orthop Clin North Am.* 2002;33:367-374.
4. Ozgur BM, Aryan HE, Pimenta L, et al. Extreme lateral interbody fusion (XLIF): a novel surgical technique for anterior lumbar interbody fusion. *Spine.* 2006;6:435-443.

SECTION IV

SPINAL INSTRUMENTATION

11

I HAVE MANY PATIENTS IN MY OFFICE WHO HAVE SYMPTOMATIC SPINAL STENOSIS. IN THE SETTING OF A LUMBAR LAMINECTOMY, WHEN SHOULD I PERFORM A FUSION?

Alpesh A. Patel, MD

First, go back a step. Surgical intervention can be divided into 2 steps: (1) neurological decompression and (2) spinal stabilization. It has been well documented that lumbar decompression is an effective procedure for symptomatic spinal stenosis. Care must be taken to obtain a thorough decompression, especially within the lateral recess. When successful, lumbar decompression has been shown to improve patient outcomes with as much success as total joint arthroplasty.[1] However, the need for surgical stabilization is much more controversial.

Spinal fusion is generally indicated in situations of instability, pathologic motion, or deformity. This is most commonly seen in patients with spondylolisthesis, scoliosis, and kyphosis. In addition, you have to keep in mind that the surgical decompression may create an iatrogenic instability or worsen a pre-existing spinal condition. Postoperative spinal instability can produce mechanical symptoms and can diminish the dimensions of the spinal canal, lateral recess, and neural foramen. This can lead to persistent or recurrent leg or back pain that, in some cases, may require a secondary surgical procedure.[2]

With this in mind, it is clear that spinal fusion should be performed when there is a concern for spinal instability. Scoliotic and kyphotic deformities have been shown to worsen after spinal decompression, leading to significant pain. I strongly consider adding a spinal fusion in this setting with the goal of preventing a progression of the deformity. The length of the fusion necessary is determined by the size and flexibility of the scoliotic or kyphotic deformity.

Degenerative spondylolisthesis is another common presentation of patients with symptomatic lumbar stenosis. Spondylolisthesis can be visualized and graded on plain radiographs. I additionally use flexion and extension lateral radiographs to determine the amount of motion present at the spondylolisthesis. In many cases, especially with significant disc space collapse, the deformity may show very little or no motion. Despite this, patients treated with fusion fair significantly better than those treated with decompression alone.[3] In most cases, therefore, I would suggest adding a fusion to limit the potential for postoperative instability, reduce the rate of recurrent symptoms, and improve overall outcomes.

References

1. Hozack WJ, Rothman RH, Albert TJ, Balderston RA, Eng K. Relationship of total hip arthroplasty outcomes to other orthopaedic procedures. *Clin Orthop Relat Res.* 1997;344:88-93.
2. Simmons ED. Surgical treatment of patients with lumbar spinal stenosis with associated scoliosis. *Clin Orthop Relat Res.* 2001;384:45-53.
3. Herkowitz HN, Kurz LT. Degenerative lumbar spondylolisthesis with spinal stenosis: a prospective study comparing decompression with decompression and intertransverse process arthrodesis. *J Bone Joint Surg Am.* 1991;73(6):802-808.

WHAT IS THE DIFFERENCE BETWEEN A POSTERIOR LUMBAR INTERBODY FUSION VERSUS A TRANSFORAMINAL INTERBODY FUSION?

Alpesh A. Patel, MD

First let's discuss the similarities. Both posterior lumbar interbody fusion (PLIF) and transforaminal interbody fusion (TLIF) approach the intervertebral disc space through a posterior spinal approach; this is in contrast to an anterior lumbar interbody fusion (ALIF). They are both typically done in addition to a posterior lumbar decompression and instrumented fusion. PLIF and TLIF, although performed for a variety of clinical indications, are surgical techniques with a common goal of improving spinal fusion rates.[1] In addition, they can be used to restore disc space height, improve sagittal balance, and indirectly decompress the neural foramen.[2]

The primary difference between the two procedures is the path of access to the intervertebral disc space (Figure 12-1). The PLIF procedure involves working in the interlaminar space with retraction of the traversing nerve root and dura to gain access to the disc space. This is typically performed on both sides of the dura with placement of a structural interbody spacer as well as bone graft. The TLIF procedure is performed through the foramen of the symptomatic side. This technique involves resection of the cranial facet as well as portions of the caudal facet articulation. After cauterization of the epidural veins, the intervertebral disc can be accessed. The TLIF approach does not require retraction of the traversing nerve root, the exiting nerve root, or the dura. In addition, a TLIF is typically performed unilaterally with the placement of a structural interbody spacer and bone graft.

A disadvantage of the PLIF technique is that it involves more significant retraction on the neural structures than TLIF. As such, neural injury, radicular pain, and dural injury have been reported more frequently with a PLIF than a TLIF.[3,4] However, there are no studies directly comparing the two procedures. In addition, there have been no reported differences in fusion or functional outcomes. Given the potential risks associated with dural retraction, I prefer to perform a TLIF in situations where I feel that posterior interbody fusion is needed (Figures 12-2 and 12-3).

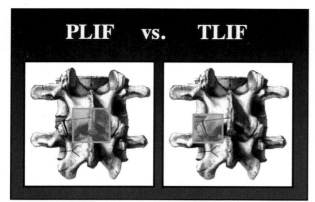

Figure 12-1. Schematic demonstrating the working windows for a TLIF versus a PLIF.

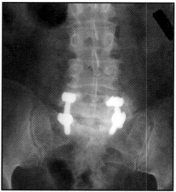

Figure 12-2. A lumbar radiograph demonstrating a TLIF cage and pedicle screws at L5-S1.

Figure 12-3. Lateral lumbar radiograph demonstrating TLIF with correction of sagittal alignment and intervertebral height restoration.

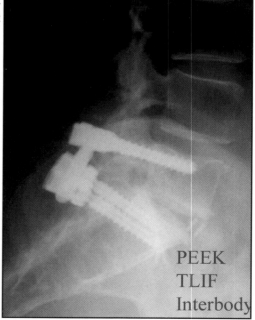

References

1. Dehoux E, Fourati E, Madi K, Reddy B, Segal P. Posterolateral versus interbody fusion in isthmic spondylolisthesis: functional results in 52 cases with a minimum follow-up of 6 years. *Acta Orthop Belg.* 2004;70(6):578-582.
2. Madan S, Boeree NR. Outcome of posterior lumbar interbody fusion versus posterolateral fusion for spondylolytic spondylolisthesis. *Spine.* 2002;27(14):1536-1542.
3. Fenton JJ, Mirza SK, Lahad A, Stern BD, Deyo RA. Variation in reported safety of lumbar interbody fusion: influence of industrial sponsorship and other study characteristics. *Spine.* 2007;32(4):471-480.
4. Anand N, Hamilton JF, Perri B, Miraliakbar H, Goldstein T. Cantilever TLIF with structural allograft and RhBMP2 for correction and maintenance of segmental sagittal lordosis: long-term clinical, radiographic, and functional outcome. *Spine.* 2006;31(20):E748-753.

13

I Have Noticed That When I Do Long Segment Fusions to the Sacrum, My Screws Have Pulled Out of the S1 Pedicle. I Am Not Familiar With Pelvic Fixation Techniques. When Should I Fuse to the Pelvis and What Types of Fixation Are Available?

Alpesh A. Patel, MD

It is often necessary to extend fusions to the sacrum in a number of patients. However, fusions to the sacrum have resulted in lumbosacral pseudarthrosis with failure of the sacral pedicle screws in a number of studies. There are two options available to improve L5-S1 fusion: anterior interbody support and posterior pelvic fixation.

The addition of pelvic fixation to a lumbosacral construct improves biomechanical stability.[1] Although the addition of an anterior cage does further restrict motion, only iliac fixation has been shown to prevent failure of sacral screws in biomechanical testing.[2] Specifically, in lumbosacral fusions extending above the L2 level, only iliac fixation has been shown to diminish strain on sacral screws. Iliac fixation should therefore be strongly considered in fusions extending from above L2 to the sacrum.

Iliac fixation options include transilieal rods, Galveston rods, and iliac screws. Unpublished data has described transileal fixation as providing excellent fusion rates with minimal complications, but it has not been widely utilized. The Galveston rod technique involves placement of rods into the pelvis, between the inner and outer cortical tables; these rods are connected to the spine proximally by wires, hooks, or screws. The Galveston technique does not provide strong iliac fixation and has been shown to loosen and fail.[3]

Iliac screw fixation has largely replaced the Galveston technique. Iliac screws are placed in a similar trajectory and provide strong fixation to the pelvis. Anatomic studies

Figure 13-1. An AP radiograph demonstrating double iliac screw fixation in the setting of a deep lumbar spine infection.

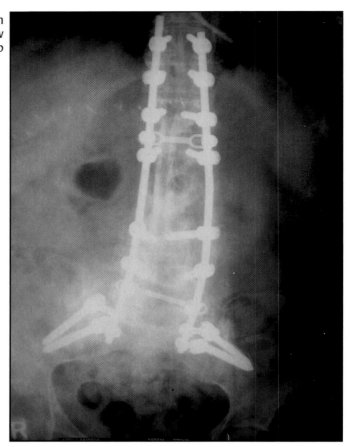

have shown that screws up to 10 mm in diameter and 141 mm in length can be placed in males, whereas screws up to 9 mm in diameter and 129 mm in length can be placed in females[4] (Figure 13-1). These can be easily connected to a lumbosacral screw/rod construct. The most common complication, reported in up to 34% of patients, is painful, prominent iliac screws requiring removal.[5]

References

1. McCord DH, Cunningham BW, Shono Y, Myers JJ, McAfee PC. Biomechanical analysis of lumbosacral fixation. *Spine*. 1992;17(8 Suppl):S235-243.
2. Cunningham BW, Lewis SJ, Long J, Dmitriev AE, Linville DA, Bridwell KH. Biomechanical evaluation of lumbosacral reconstruction techniques for spondylolisthesis: an in-vitro porcine model. *Spine*. 2002;27(21):2321-2327.
3. Peelle MW, Lenke LG, Bridwell KH, Sides B. Comparison of pelvic fixation techniques in neuromuscular spinal deformity correction: Galveston rod versus iliac and lumbosacral screws. *Spine*. 2006;31(20):2392-2398; discussion 2399.
4. Schildhauer TA, McCulloch P, Chapman JR, Mann FA. Anatomic and radiographic considerations for placement of transiliac screws in lumbopelvic fixations. *J Spinal Disord Tech*. 2002;15(3):199-205; discussion 205.
5. Tsuchiya K, Bridwell KH, Kuklo TR, Lenke LG, Baldus C. Minimum 5-year analysis of L5-S1 fusion using sacropelvic fixation (bilateral S1 and iliac screws) for spinal deformity. *Spine*. 2006;31(3):303-308.

14

I HAVE A 34-YEAR-OLD MALE WHO HAS DEGENERATIVE DISC DISEASE AT L4-5 AND WANTS TO AVOID A FUSION. WHAT ARE THE ADVANTAGES AND DISADVANTAGES OF A LUMBAR DISC REPLACEMENT IN A YOUNG INDIVIDUAL?

Alpesh A. Patel, MD

First, I would strongly advise reconsidering surgical intervention of any kind in a young patient with axial back pain and no neurological symptoms. The outcomes are not as good for the treatment of back pain in isolation as they are for neurological symptoms. In patients with level 1 degenerative disc disease, I would exhaust all options including physical therapy, medications, and injections prior to surgical intervention. Although controversial, I would then use lumbar discography to confirm that the level of concern is the only concordant pain generator. If any other sources of pain (another spinal level, sacroiliac joints) are identified, I would not recommend surgery.

If a single degenerative level is identified as the source of pain and the patient has failed all other measures, I would consider either a fusion or a lumbar arthroplasty (Figures 14-1 to 14-3). The potential advantages to lumbar disc arthroplasty are only theoretical at this time: motion preservation and prevention of adjacent level degeneration and disease. Studies have shown that motion after lumbar arthroplasty can average 10 degrees of flexion/extension and 5 degrees of lateral motion.[1] However, other studies have demonstrated that excellent pain relief can be obtained even with complete ankylosis of the disc arthroplasty.[2] The importance of motion preservation is therefore in question.

Adjacent level disease, defined as symptomatic degeneration, can lead to a recurrence of pain and neurologic symptoms after lumbar fusion and can require further surgery. We believe that adjacent level disease is due to the altered mechanical properties of the lumbar spine after fusion. In contrast, the recreation of physiologic biomechanics in the

Figure 14-1. Diagramatic representation of the relationship of the anterior neural and vascular structures at the L5-S1 disc space.

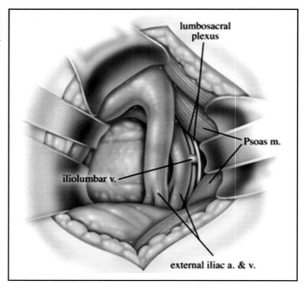

lumbar spine with disc arthroplasty should reduce the development of adjacent level degeneration. However, the incidence of adjacent level disease after lumbar arthroplasty has yet to be well defined through prospective studies.

In contrast, we know of many potential disadvantages associated with lumbar arthroplasty. Primarily, disc arthroplasty requires an anterior approach to the spine. There is documented risk of vascular injury (3.6%) as well as retrograde ejaculation after anterior spinal surgery[3] (Figure 14-1). Additionally, in the United States, many insurance providers will not approve arthroplasty, leaving the patient with a large financial debt.

We also know that failure of the lumbar arthroplasty is a distinct possibility. This occurs most commonly through either errors in patient selection or surgical technique. Lumbar arthroplasty is contraindicated if spondylolisthesis or degenerative facet arthrosis is present. In addition, inappropriate implant sizing and positioning have led to early arthroplasty failure. Later failures resulting from implant migration or polyethylene failure have been noted.

Perhaps the most daunting disadvantage of lumbar arthroplasty is the possible need for revision surgery. Revision is needed in 8 to 11% of cases in large arthroplasty studies.[2,3] Treatment options involving explantation of the arthroplasty device require a revised anterior surgical approach. Vascular injury has been reported in 16% of revised arthroplasty cases, in some cases with life-threatening results.[3] In addition, we know that the risk of ureteral injury and retrograde ejaculation is higher in revised cases. Although techniques to reduce abdominal adhesions have been proposed, there is no data to show that they reduce these risks (Figures 14-2 and 14-3).

At this time, therefore, I would strongly consider avoiding surgery altogether or to consider a lumbar arthrodesis. Once data is available to show superiority of lumbar arthroplasty over lumbar arthrodesis, then disc arthroplasty may be a more viable option.

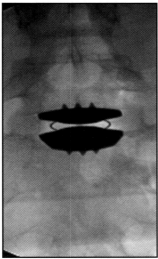

Figure 14-2. AP fluoroscope image of a disc arthroplasty demonstrating a midline placement.

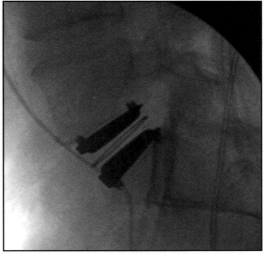

Figure 14-3. Lateral fluoroscopic image demonstrating appropriate placement of the disc arthroplasty at the L5-S1 level.

References

1. Lemaire JP, Carrier H, Sariali el H, Skalli W, Lavaste F. Clinical and radiological outcomes with the Charite artificial disc: a 10-year minimum follow-up. *J Spinal Disord Tech*. 2005;18(4):353-359.
2. Putzier M, Funk JF, Schneider SV, et al. Charite total disc replacement--clinical and radiographical results after an average follow-up of 17 years. *Eur Spine J*. 2006;15(2):183-195.
3. McAfee PC, Geisler FH, Saiedy SS, et al. Revisability of the CHARITE artificial disc replacement: analysis of 688 patients enrolled in the U.S. IDE study of the CHARITE Artificial Disc. *Spine*. 2006;31(11):1217-1226.

SECTION V

TUMOR

15

I HAVE A 37-YEAR-OLD MALE WITH AN ISOLATED LYTIC BONE LESION IN HIS THORACIC VERTEBRA. HIS BIOPSY INDICATED A GIANT CELL TUMOR. HOW DO I MANAGE THIS LESION?

Alpesh A. Patel, MD

I would make sure that the patient understands the pathology surrounding giant cell tumors (GCT) well. GCTs are described as benign but locally aggressive lesions that typically occur in males between 20 and 50 years of age. In the spine, they present as painful lytic lesions in the vertebral body with neurological deficits in some patients. The most common differential diagnoses in this age group includes nonossifying fibroma, aneurismal bone cysts, metastatic disease, multiple myeloma, infection, and brown tumors associated with hyperparathyroidism. Before the biopsy occurred, I would have obtained complete spine radiographs as well as a skeletal survey to identify other lesions that may be present. This would help with the differential diagnosis. Additionally, in a younger patient, there is a possibility, albeit rare, of multifocal GCT. I would also have obtained an MRI of the spine to assist with staging of the lesion. Specifically, I would try to evaluate any extracortical extension of the tumor mass as this will change treatment options. The MRI would also identify other lesions that may not be visualized on routine radiographs. Laboratory studies can also be obtained, prior to biopsy, to help with the differential diagnosis. Serum and urine protein electrophoresis can define a plasmacytoma or multiple myeloma in lieu of a tissue biopsy.

At this point, we now have a tissue diagnosis of GCT (Figure 15-1). We must remember that brown tumors associated with hyperparathyroidism can produce a pattern histologically similar to GCT. I would check serum calcium and parathyroid levels to rule out hyperparathyroidism. In the next step, I would obtain a CT scan of the patient's chest to identify pulmonary metastases that may be present (Figure 15-2). Although GCT is

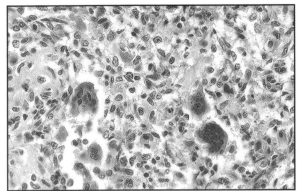

Figure 15-1. Histological section demonstrating the presence of multiple multi-nucleated cells (giant cells).

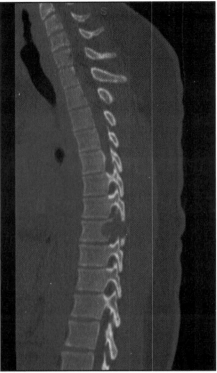

Figure 15-3. Sagittal CT scan demonstrating recurrence of the giant cell with extension into the spinal canal. (Image courtesy of James Harrop, MD, Department of Neurosurgery, Thomas Jefferson University, Phiadelphia, PA.)

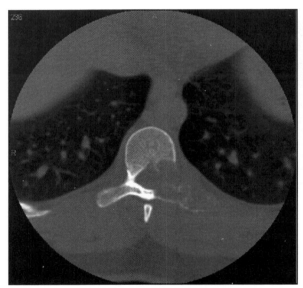

Figure 15-2. Axial CT scan image demonstrating lytic destruction of the vertebral body and right pedicle. (Image courtesy of James Harrop, MD, Department of Neurosurgery, Thomas Jefferson University, Phiadelphia, PA.)

described as histologically benign, it is known to recur locally in 10 to 30% of patients and lead to pulmonary metastases in an about 5% of patients.[1] Although these metastatic foci are histologically similar to the primary site, they can lead to death in up to 25% of individuals.[2] Because of this, I would strongly recommend excision of metastatic pulmonary lesions when possible.

The treatment of the vertebral lesion is based upon its staging, the presence of metastatic disease, and the presence of neurologic compression. The staging strategy described for GCT is broken into three stages. Stage 1 lesions are considered latent with no evidence

locally aggressive with significant changes in the cortical bone or with evidence of tumor penetration through the cortex.

Stage 1 and stage 2 lesions can be treated with intralesional excision through an open curettage and bone graft technique. You need to be sure to remove all tissue from within the tumor cavity, including the pseudocaspule. This may be augmented with adjunctive agents such as phenol or polymethlymethacrylate to eliminate any tumors that may be present in small crevasses that are otherwise hard to visualize. In the thoracic spine, I would do this either through a thoracotomy or a video-assisted thoracoscopy. Because of the caustic properties of phenol, I would not advise using it in the thoracic cavity. Percutaneous placement of polymethlymethacrylate has been described in a case report, but I would not use this as my primary treatment option.[3]

Stage 3 lesions, any patient demonstrating malignant changes on biopsy, any patient with metastatic disease, any patient with neurologic compression, and any patient with a recurrent lesion should be treated with an extralesional resection with as much margin of healthy tissue as possible.

In this patient, the lesion would be defined as stage 3. I would perform an en bloc spondylectomy of the involved segment. If the tumor mass has an extracortical component, I would be sure to remove the tumor around its pseudocapsule in an attempt to avoid tumor spillage. After tumor excision, I would reconstruct the spine with an iliac crest autograft, which should be obtained through a separate incision prior to the tumor resection. Allograft bone or use of an expandable cage are other options; however, I feel that autograft bone affords the best healing rate. In addition, the presence of a metallic cage may make detection of tumor recurrence very difficult. I would typically reinforce the anterior reconstruction with a posterior instrumented fusion, although stand-alone anterior reconstruction is another option in the thoracic spine.

I would avoid the use of adjuvant radiation therapy in most cases. In cases with extra-cortical tumor extension, with tumor spillage during resection, or with evidence of meta-static disease, the use of postoperative radiation therapy is more controversial. There is little data to show improved survival or reduced recurrence rates.

Lastly, these patients need to be monitored for well past 5 to 10 years because recurrence rates can be quite high (Figure 15-3). I would recommend restaging all patients (MRI scan, plain radiographs, CT scan of chest) who have a recurrence of pain symptoms after surgery. In patients with an intralesional curettage, I would obtain CT scans on a yearly basis to detect any early recurrence.

References

1. Sanjay BK, Sim FH, Unni KK, McLeod RA, Klassen RA. Giant-cell tumours of the spine. *J Bone Joint Surg Br.* 1993;75(1):148-154.
2. Rock MG, Pritchard DJ, Unni KK. Metastases from histologically benign giant-cell tumor of bone. *J Bone Joint Surg Am.* 1984;66(2):269-274.
3. Paul L, Santonja C, Izquierdo E. Complete necrosis of a spinal giant cell tumor after vertebroplasty. *J Vasc Interv Radiol.* 2006;17(4):727-731.

16

I Have an Elderly Patient With Multiple Lesions in the Cervical/Thoracic and Lumbar Spine. Which Laboratory and Imaging Studies Should I Obtain?

Alpesh A. Patel, MD

At the initial assessment, I would obtain full spinal radiographs as well as a complete skeletal survey to assess other bony lesions that may be present. The presence of multiple lytic lesions in an elderly patient would most commonly suggest either metastatic disease or multiple myeloma. Both disease processes can affect the axial and appendicular skeleton. Early detection and treatment of long bone or hip lesions may prevent a pathological fracture.

The patient's history, such as cigarette smoking, may point toward a primary tumor. A thorough physical exam of the patient, including examination of the breast (females predominately), prostate (males), and lymphatic system is needed to help detect a primary tumor source. Cancer screening exams, such as mammography and colonoscopy, should also be performed if needed. In addition to this, I would obtain CT scans of the patient's head, chest, abdomen, and pelvis. This may identify metastatic tumors present within other organ systems such as the liver, lungs, and central nervous system that may help identify a primary tumor site such as the lung, kidneys, large bowel, ovaries, or pancreas.

A standard Technitium-99 (Tc^{99}) radionucleotide bone scan may demonstrate skeletal lesions that are otherwise not visualized on routine radiographs. Bone scans highlight areas of high bone turnover, specifically areas of high osteoblastic function. Most metastatic tumors lead to bone turnover through a paracrine effect on native osteoclasts, which secondarily activate osteoblasts. Multiple myeloma, in contrast, directly causes bony destruction, avoiding the osteoclastic/osteoblastic pathway. A bone scan in multiple myeloma lesions is therefore notoriously "cold" in a large number of patients. Therefore,

I do not rely on standard Tc^{99} bone scans to identify all multiple myeloma lesions. Although modifications of standard bone scans have been demonstrated to identify and track multiple myeloma lesions, they are not widely available.[1]

I would obtain a magnetic resonance imaging (MRI) scan of the cervical, thoracic, and lumbar spine to evaluate the known lesions as well as to identify lesions that may not be seen on routine imaging or radionucleotide scans.[2] Although the MRI will not help with the differential diagnosis, it provides anatomic information as to the size and location of the lesions as well as any neurological compression that may also exist. This is invaluable information when the time comes to decide on the treatment.

Laboratory studies can aid in the diagnosis of both metastatic disease and multiple myeloma. Serum erythrocyte sedimentation rate will be elevated in both diseases. Serum alkaline phosphatase is typically elevated in metastatic disease because of high osteoblastic activity. Again, because of the direct effect of multiple myeloma on bone destruction, alkaline phosphatase is usually not elevated in multiple myeloma. I do not rely heavily on alkaline phosphatase because a number of disease processes can affect serum levels; it is most useful in cases of Paget's disease.

Serum protein electrophoresis (SPEP) will typically identify a discrete, abnormal band of immunoglobulin (IgA or IgG) in 80 to 90% of patients. Major criteria for diagnosis include a monoclonal globulin spike larger than 3.5 g (for IgG) or larger than 2.0 g (for IgA) per 100 ml. In addition, urine protein electrophoresis (UPEP) can identify a monoclonal spike in 50% of patients, especially those with an IgG myeloma.[2] Evidence of anemia, thrombocytopenia, renal failure, or hypercalcemia points to multiple myeloma. The anemia is usually a normocytic, normochromic anemia with Hct results of less than 30%. Renal failure is due to the nephrotoxicity of the IgG lambda light chains. Hypercalcemia, due to renal failure, is seen in up to 40% of patients with multiple myeloma.

References

1. Koutsikos J, Grigoraki V, Athanasoulis T, et al. Scintigraphy with technetium-99m methoxyisobutylisonitrile in multiple myeloma patients: correlation with the International Staging System. *Hell J Nucl Med.* 2006;9(3):177-180.
2. Zamagni E, Nanni C, Patriarca F, et al. A prospective comparison of 18F-fluorodeoxyglucose positron emission tomography-computed tomography, magnetic resonance imaging and whole-body planar radiographs in the assessment of bone disease in newly diagnosed multiple myeloma. *Haematologica.* 2007;92(1):50-55.
3. O'Connell TX, Horita TJ, Kasravi B. Understanding and interpreting serum protein electrophoresis. *Am Fam Physician.* 2005;71(1):105-112.

I Have a 67-Year-Old Female with Metastatic Breast Cancer and Spinal Cord Compression in the Thoracic Spine. When Should I Perform Surgery Instead of Irradiation?

Alpesh A. Patel, MD

I would consider surgical treatment in all patients with metastatic spinal column disease and spinal cord compression with neurologic symptoms. If the patient has no neurological symptoms, you can consider radiation treatment, because breast cancer can be locally amenable to radiation treatment.

Spinal cord compression has been reported to occur in up to 20% of patients with metastatic cancer, most commonly in the thoracic spine. Traditional thinking in managing these patients has been to avoid surgical intervention. The life span of many of these patients can be limited, and as such surgery has been thought of as aggressive. With this in mind, steroid treatment and radiation therapy are often initially prescribed.

Treatment with steroids can been effective for spinal cord compression associated with lymphoma; in other patients, however, there have been no reported benefits in neurological recovery or survival. External beam radiation therapy is another treatment option that has been described. Radiation therapy has been shown to improve neurological function in up to 40% of patients with radiosensitive tumors such as myeloma, lymphoma, and breast cancer.[1] However, it has not been shown to improve survival and has been reported to increase the risk of pathological fracture. In addition, a number of common tumors (thyroid, renal cell, lung) are resistant to radiation treatment.

In sharp contrast, a number of studies have shown that surgical treatment improves neurological function across a wide array of tumor types. Surgical options include posterior decompression, posterior decompression and stabilization, anterior decompression and stabilization, and combined anterior and posterior procedures. Posterior decompression alone has demonstrated an improvement in 44% of patients on average, with mortality in up to 7% of patients. I would therefore strongly recommend against a posterior decompression procedure.

The addition of surgical stabilization through instrumentation as well as structural bone grafts has significantly improved outcomes. Posterior decompression and stabilization has been reported to improve neurological function in 67% of patients on average, with an 8% mortality rate. Direct decompression of the anterior compressive tumor mass has shown even better results, with an average of 76% patients demonstrating neurological improvement, although the mortality rate is slightly higher at 10%.

These studies have demonstrated that surgical decompression and stabilization is much more effective at improving neurological function in patients but have not demonstrated improved survival or discussed functional outcomes. However, a recent pivotal study demonstrated both improvements in functional outcomes (ambulation, continence) and survival.[2] In a prospective study of patients with metastatic spinal cord compression, subjects were randomized to radiation treatment or early surgical decompression and stabilization with postoperative radiation. This study demonstrated such superiority in ambulation, continence, and survival in the surgical group that the study was terminated early. Most impressively, among patients who lost the ability to walk, 56% in the surgical group but only 19% in the radiation group regained the ability to ambulate. In addition, those patients who were first in the radiation group and then crossed over to the surgical group showed poorer results and higher complications than patients initially treated surgically.

With this data in mind, I consider surgical intervention in all patients with metastatic spinal cord compression and neurological symptoms. I will typically perform an anterior column decompression, through an anterior approach or through a posterior costotransversectomy, with reconstruction of the anterior column using an allograft or an expandable cage. I will supplement this with a posterior instrumented fusion. I would delay radiation therapy for at least 2 to 3 weeks to prevent wound complications in the postoperative period. Once the incision has healed, I will use an external beam radiotherapy protocol as a postoperative adjunct to surgical decompression.

References

1. Constans JP, de Divitiis E, Donzelli, R, Spaziante R, Meder JE, Haye C. Spinal metastases with neurological manifestations: review of 600 cases. *J Neurosurg.* 1983; 59(1): 111-118.
2. Patchell RA, Tibbs PA, Regine WF, et al. Direct decompressive surgical resection in the treatment of spinal cord compression caused by metastatic cancer: a randomised trial. *Lancet.* 2005;366(9486):643-648.

SECTION VI

INFECTION

WHAT RISK FACTORS WILL INCREASE THE LIKELIHOOD OF POSTOPERATIVE INFECTION?

Ahmad Nassr, MD and Joon Y. Lee, MD

The incidence of infection after primary spine surgery can vary from 1 to 12%.[1] Preoperative risk factors correlating with infection include advanced age, diabetes, obesity, heavy alcohol use, previous lumbar surgery, current or history of previous infection, and smoking. Intraoperative risk factors for infection include prolonged operative time, staged anterior/posterior procedures, and procedures with increased blood loss. Specifically, Fang et al retrospectively reviewed more than 1629 spinal procedures performed in 1095 patients and identified 48 cases of infection, an infection rate of 4.4%.[2] This study also identified age greater than 60, smoking, diabetes, obesity, alcohol abuse, and a history of previous spinal infection as significant risk factors for spinal infection.

Immunocompromised patients are especially prone to postoperative wound infections. This group includes patients afflicted with immunosuppressive disease (ie, AIDS), patients under medically induced immunosupression (ie, organ transplant and rheumatoid patients), and those with nutritional deficiencies. Patients with nutritional deficiency should have full nutritional consultation and treatment prior to surgery. Patients using antirheumatic agents should consider temporary cessation of these medications, although this may be controversial. If the rheumatologist and patient are comfortable stopping these medications for a time both before and after surgery and doing so would not significantly risk aggravating the rheumatoid arthritis, then it is probably wise to do this, given the sometimes devastating effects of a postoperative infection.

Patients who have had organ transplants usually cannot stop the immunosuppressants pre- or postoperatively. Although the exact rate of postoperative infection is not known, these patients are particularly at risk for a fulminate infection or sepsis if a wound infection were to occur. This risk should be discussed in detail with the patient before the operation.

One of the most frequently encountered risk factors is diabetes. Some evidence suggests blood glucose levels in the postoperative period that are greater than 200 mg/dl predispose patients to wound infections. Postoperative blood glucose control has also been shown to be an independent risk factor for infection after vascular surgeries as well. Some surgeons have advocated the use of a perioperative insulin drip protocol for more precise control of blood glucose levels. We recommend an endocrine consultation for all diabetic patients to aid in stringent blood glucose control.

The use of preoperative antibiotics has been shown to clearly decrease the rate of postoperative infection in elective surgery. This is especially true if the antibiotics are given 2 hours prior to the skin incision. Pre- and perioperative antibiotics have been used as part of protocols designed to decrease the incidence of postoperative infection after spine surgery. We use preoperative antibiotics given at the induction of anesthesia, which are redosed every 3 to 4 hours during the operation and continued postoperatively for 24 hours to decrease the risk of infection.

References

1. Beiner JM, Grauer J, Kwon BK, et al. Postoperative wound infections of the spine. *Neurosurg Focus.* 2003;15: E14.
2. Fang A, Hu SS, Endres N, et al. Risk factors for infection after spinal surgery. *Spine.* 2005;30:1460-1465.

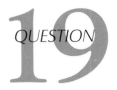

QUESTION

19

I Have a Patient Who Has a Draining Wound 2 Weeks After a Lumbar Laminectomy Fusion. How Should I Manage This Patient? What if the Patient Had This Infection 9 Months Later?

Ahmad Nassr, MD and Joon Y. Lee, MD

Patients presenting with a draining wound more than 2 weeks after surgery should be treated for a probable infection. Several studies have shown that prolonged wound drainage is associated with an increased risk of infection.[1] We treat these patients with an operative debridement with the assumption of a deep infection (Figure 19-1). The wound should be opened and all superficial sutures removed because these are sources of retained bacteria. Superficial tissue and fluid samples should be sent for aerobic, anaerobic, and fungal cultures as well as for pathology. The superficial wound should be debrided of any nonviable tissue, followed by pulsatile-lavage irrigation of the superficial wound. Only once the superficial wound is cleaned should the deep fascia be opened. Irrigation of the deep wound should also be performed using pulse lavage, taking care to retain the previous bone graft as long as it does not appear to be grossly infected and/or loose (Figure 19-2).

If instrumentation is present, we retain the hardware in the setting of an acute infection because it provides stability for the fusion. The fascia is then closed over a deep suction drain, preferably with an absorbable monofilament suture. The decision to close the skin primarily, allow healing by secondary intention, or use a vacuum-assisted wound-closure device depends on the severity of the infection. Patients with relatively mild drainage and without gross purulence may be closed primarily with the placement of multiple drains (we prefer Jackson-Pratt drains). These drains should be left in place until drainage is minimal. Those patients with gross purulence should undergo multiple irrigation and debridement procedures every 48 to 72 hours until definitive closure. If the wound continues to appear purulent after multiple irrigation and debridement procedures, or primary closure is difficult, vacuum-assisted closure (VAC) should be considered.

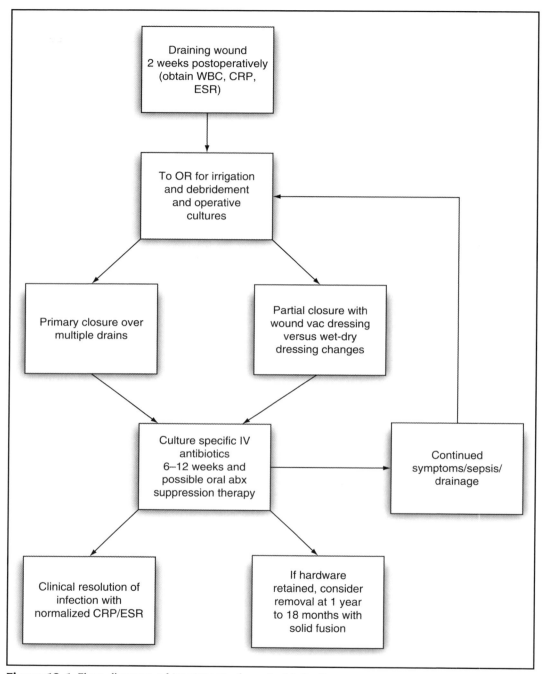

Figure 19-1. Flow diagram of treatment of surgical infection.

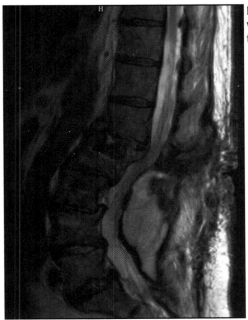

Figure 19-2. MRI study of deep wound infection. T2 weighted image shows collection of fluid deep in the fascia during the acute postoperative period.

VAC may be helpful in patients with an impaired wound, including the malnourished and elderly. The VAC sponge is placed on top of the fascia after a partial wound closure. VAC can be used with good results even in more complex wounds where exposed hardware is present. The advantages of the VAC device over the traditional wet-to-dry dressing changes are faster wound healing and the convenience of less frequent dressing changes.

In all cases, we place patients on broad-spectrum intravenous antibiotics while cultures are pending. An infectious disease consultation should be obtained. A peripherally inserted central venous catheter should be inserted in anticipation of 6 to 12 weeks of culture-specific antibiotics. Serial measurements of WBC count, erythrocyte sedimentation rate (ESR), and C-reactive protein (CRP) should be performed to monitor the response of the infection to the antibiotic regimen. We tend to rely upon the CRP as a measure of response to treatment because it has been clinically correlated.[2] The ESR can sometimes remain elevated even in the face of clinical improvement.[2] Recurrent drainage or signs of systemic illness should prompt the surgeon to consider repeated operative debridement. If tissue coverage of the existing instrumentation is not possible, plastic surgical consultation for flap coverage should be considered.

References

1. Beiner JM, Grauer J, Kwon BK, et al. Postoperative wound infections of the spine. *Neurosurg Focus.* 2003;15: E14.
2. Khan MH, Smith PN, Rao N, et al. Serum C-reactive protein levels correlate with clinical response in patients treated with antibiotics for wound infections after spinal surgery. *Spine.* 2006;6:311-315.

SECTION VII

TRAUMA

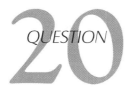

QUESTION

20

I HAVE A 28-YEAR-OLD FEMALE WITH A T12 BURST FRACTURE. SHE IS NEUROLOGICALLY INTACT WITH 40 DEGREES OF KYPHOSIS AND 50% CANAL COMPROMISE. CAN I DO AN ALL-POSTERIOR FUSION OR SHOULD I PLAN ON GOING ANTERIORLY?

Ahmad Nassr, MD and Joon Y. Lee, MD

The treatment algorithm of neurologically intact patients with unstable burst fractures of the thoraco-lumbar spine is controversial. One debate centers on whether operative management is superior to nonoperative management. Given that this patient has a significant kyphosis (40 degrees) and 50% canal compromise, one can assume that this injury has a high likelihood of collapsing further. Preoperative CT and magnetic resonance imaging (MRI) can be helpful in determining the stability of an injury. CT scans may reveal the severity of the burst fracture with the loss of anterior and middle columns. MRI may indicate loss of posterior stabilizing complexes (interspinous ligament, ligamentum flavum, and joint capsules), which allow the fracture to fall into kyphosis. If these signs are present, then we would recommend operative management. The method of reconstruction, whether it is performed anteriorly, posteriorly, or both, is a matter of debate.

The combination of anterior decompression and arthrodesis has been shown to be a safe and effective procedure in the treatment of unstable burst fractures. It has the advantage of being able to decompress the spinal canal, especially if there is a neurologic injury, and provide fixation without the need and morbidity of a posterior fusion. Sasso et al studied 40 patients, who showed an apparent fusion rate of 95%.[1] In this group of patients, the average preoperative kyphosis was 22.7 degrees and was corrected to 7.4 degrees with the surgery. They reported a loss of only 2.1 degrees of correction at latest follow-up.

A posterior-only construct is a viable option for a neurologically intact patient and obviates the morbidity of an anterior approach.

Short-segment posterior constructs for unstable fractures including only one level above and below the fracture have been attempted to spare motion segments in the lumbar spine. These constructs, however, have a high failure rate because of the lack of anterior structural support, which results in posterior construct failure. In a prospective study by Tezeren et al, 18 patients were randomized into either short-segment or traditional long-fixation groups.[2] The short-segment fixation group had a 55% failure rate with a significant loss of correction. Traditional long-fixation constructs (Figure 20-1) were better at maintaining correction. However, there was no significant difference in their clinical outcomes. In more traditional constructs, two levels above and below the injury level are included in the fusion. In either case, a postural

Figure 20-1. Twenty-eight year-old female who underwent an extracavitary corpectomy and posterior spinal fusion with an expandable cage from an all-posterior approach.

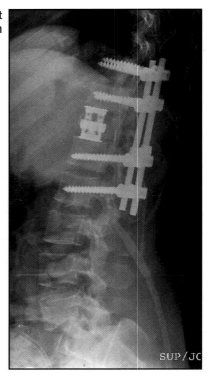

reduction by positioning on a Jackson table is performed and then ligamentotaxis is used to partially decompress the spinal canal.

In combined surgical approaches, the anterior approach is performed to decompress the spinal canal, and then reconstruction is performed using either a structural allograft or prosthetic device. This can then be followed by posterior instrumentation. This has the advantage of providing anterior structural support, which allows for load sharing with the posterior instrumentation and thereby decreases the likelihood of kyphosis. Biomechanical testing has demonstrated the superiority of combined approaches when compared to isolated anterior-only or posterior-only approaches.[3]

If the imaging studies support posterior ligamentous complex injury (injury to interspinous ligament, ligamentum flavum, or joint capsules), we would consider combined anterior and posterior reconstruction in this patient. Given the amount of kyphosis, there is a significant loss of anterior and middle column support that may predispose this patient to progressive kyphosis if only posterior fixation is performed. A combined approach can maximize correction and also allow reconstruction of the anterior and middle columns. The anterior reconstruction would be followed by posterior instrumented arthrodesis from T10-L1 or L2 depending upon the patient's sagittal alignment.

References

1. Sasso RC, Best NM, Reilly TM, et al. Anterior-only stabilization of three-column thoracolumbar injuries. *J Spinal Disord Tech.* 2005;18 Suppl:S7-14.
2. Tezeren G, Kuru I. Posterior fixation of thoracolumbar burst fracture: short-segment pedicle fixation versus long-segment instrumentation. *J Spinal Disord Tech.* 2005;18:485-488.
3. Wilke HJ, Kemmerich V, Claes LE, et al. Combined anteroposterior spinal fixation provides superior stabilisation to a single anterior or posterior procedure. *J Bone Joint Surg Br.* 2001;83:609-617.

WHAT SCREENING RADIOGRAPHS SHOULD A SPINAL TRAUMA PATIENT GET?

Ahmad Nassr, MD and Joon Y. Lee, MD

Several factors determine whether spine radiographs are necessary in trauma patients. These factors can vary from clinical clearance of the spine to the use of more advanced diagnostic modalities such as computer tomography (CT) and magnetic resonance imaging (MRI).[1]

In patients who are awake and cooperative with low-energy injuries and no complaints of spinal pain or neurologic dysfunction, clinical clearance of the spine can be performed reasonably well without obtaining any imaging studies. Most trauma centers rely upon an initial series of radiographs including a lateral cervical spine, anteroposterior (AP) chest, and pelvic x-rays. An adequate cervical spine x-ray is often very difficult to obtain, because it should be a nonrotated film with visualization of the occipital-cervical as well as the cervical-thoracic junctions. It is often difficult to visualize the cervical-thoracic junction, which necessitates special views such as a swimmer's view or a traction film, which may be impractical in a trauma patient. If a cervical spine injury is suspected, then the lateral x-ray should be complemented with an AP and open-mouth radiograph. With these three x-rays, the majority of cervical fractures will be identified.[2]

There is some debate about the use of flexion and extension lateral radiographs in the acute setting. There is ample literature to suggest that these may be of limited value because patients with neck injuries may have significant muscular spasms and limited range of motion, making these imaging studies of minimal value. If adequate films cannot be obtained, then a CT scan of the cervical spine through the upper thoracic spine should be obtained with sagittal and coronal reconstruction to rule out any bony injury. CT scanning should also be considered in patients who have negative radiographs but continue to complain of pain or present with a neurologic deficit (Figure 21-1).

If a cervical injury has been detected, then a CT scan with sagittal and coronal reconstructions should be obtained. This should be complemented with imaging of the thoracic

Figure 21-1. Lateral radiograph and CT scan of a patient involved in a motor vehicle collision. Patient's x-rays suggest an odontoid fracture, but this may be easily missed. In this case, a CT scan is a good study to identify the fracture.

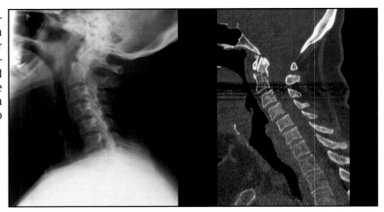

and lumbar spine because of the incidence of noncontiguous spine injuries. This can be in the form of AP and lateral radiographs or CT scanning of the thoracic and lumbar spine. Imaging of the thoraco-lumbar spine should also be obtained in patients with lap-belt injuries (bruising of the abdomen or thorax), falls from heights, or pain to palpation of the thoracic or lumbar spine during examination. Many times the same CT scan used by the trauma surgeons to evaluate the thorax and abdomen will be sufficient to evaluate the thoracic and lumbar spine.

Fractures of the sacrum can usually be identified by the AP pelvis x-ray and, if confirmed, should prompt dedicated films of the pelvis and CT of the thoraco-lumbar spine. Some trauma centers have recently advocated using spiral CT scans as means for initial assessment of the spine. CT scanning has became a quick and cost-effective means of evaluating the entire spine, and many institutions are using CT instead of plain radiographs for initial assesment.[3] Once an injury is identified, dedicated plain radiographs are obtained of the affected area because they aid in determining fracture morphology and alignment.

MRI is rarely used in the acute trauma setting because of the long acquisition time. However, there are settings where these studies become extremely valuable and can alter treatment decisions. The most frequently encountered scenario that may warrant an MRI is a cervical facet dislocation. Obtaining a pre-reduction MRI has been debated, but it can aid in the detection of a cervical disc herniation, which may necessitate an open reduction to decrease the chance of neurologic deterioration.[4]

References

1. France JC, Bono CM, Vaccaro AR. Initial radiographic evaluation of the spine after trauma: when, what, where, and how to image the acutely traumatized spine. *J Orthop Trauma.* 2005;19:640-649.
2. MacDonald RL, Schwartz ML, Mirich D, et al. Diagnosis of cervical spine injury in motor vehicle crash victims: how many X-rays are enough? *J Trauma.* 1990;30:392-397.
3. Grogan EL, Morris JA Jr, Dittus RS, et al. Cervical spine evaluation in urban trauma centers: lowering institutional costs and complications through helical CT scan. *J Am Coll Surg.* 2005;200:160-165.
4. Vaccaro AR, Zeiller SC, Hulbert RJ, et al. The thoracolumbar injury severity score: a proposed treatment algorithm. *J Spinal Disord Tech.* 2005;18:209-215.

I Have a 27-Year-Old Male With a C5-6 Facet Dislocation Who Is Awake and Alert. Do I Need to Get an MRI Before I Reduce the Facet Dislocation?

Ahmad Nassr, MD and Joon Y. Lee, MD

Reduction of a cervical facet dislocation without a pre-reduction magnetic resonance imaging (MRI) scan has been controversial. In a patient that is awake and alert, we would argue that an MRI is not necessary because the patient can cooperate with serial neurologic exams during the reduction. Serial exams are performed after the addition of any weight during the reduction process. If any neurologic deterioration is noted during the reduction, then all weight is removed and an emergent MRI is obtained.

Eismont et al described a case report of neurologic worsening after closed reduction of a patient with a cervical facet dislocation.[1] This article has prompted controversy about the safety of closed reductions without pre-reduction MRI. However, the patient described by Eismont et al received sedation during the reduction. Vaccaro et al have shown that closed reduction in an awake and cooperative patient even in the face of an apparent disk herniation can still be performed safely.[2]

An MRI obtained prior to reduction will help identify a disk herniation (Figure 22-1) or hematoma, convincing the surgeon to perform an anterior procedure to decompress the spinal cord. Pre-reduction MRIs may lead to unnecessary surgery on asymptomatic disc herniation in an awake and cooperative patient.

References

1. Eismont FJ, Arena MJ, Green BA. Extrusion of an intervertebral disc associated with traumatic subluxation or dislocation of cervical facets: case report. *J Bone Joint Surg Am.* 1991;73:1555-1560.

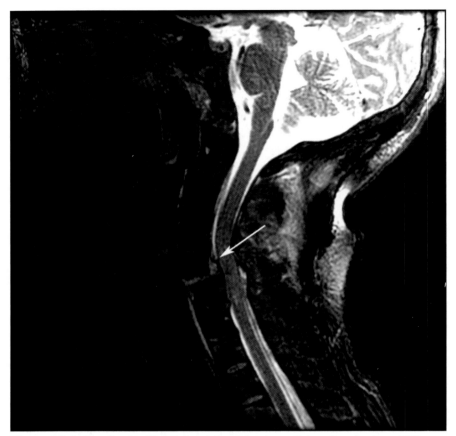

Figure 22-1. A patient with bilateral facet fracture dislocation had an MRI performed prior to reduction. The white arrow shows a disc herniation behind the vertebral body. Whether this disc will be pushed into the spinal cord or reduced into the native position during the reduction is unknown. We would argue that obtaining MRI routinely on these patients, especially if they are awake and cooperative, may lead to delay in reduction of the spine.

2. Vaccaro AR, Falatyn SP, Flanders AE, et al. Magnetic resonance evaluation of the intervertebral disc, spinal ligaments, and spinal cord before and after closed traction reduction of cervical spine dislocations. *Spine.* 1999;24:1210-1217.

QUESTION

23

WHAT IS SPINAL SHOCK?
HOW DO I KNOW WHEN IT IS OVER?

Ahmad Nassr, MD and Joon Y. Lee, MD

Spinal shock is a combination of areflexia/hyporeflexia and autonomic dysfunction that accompanies spinal cord injury. The initial hyporeflexia presents as a loss of both cutaneous and deep tendon reflexes below the level of injury accompanied by loss of sympathetic outflow, resulting in hypotension and bradycardia. Reflexes generally return in a specific pattern, with cutaneous reflexes generally returning before deep tendon reflexes.

Ko et al[1] have described a specific pattern of reflex return with the delayed plantar reflex (DPR) returning first, followed by the bulbocavernosis (BC) and cremasteric (CR) reflexes, and finally the ankle and knee jerk reflexes (AJ, KJ). As mentioned previously, the first reflex to return is an abnormal delayed plantar reflex (DPR). The second reflex that returns is the bulbocavernosous reflex (BCR). This reflex is checked to determine the ending of spinal shock. A BCR is elicited by squeezing the penile glans or the clitoris and feeling for an involuntary contraction of the anus. Tugging on a foley catheter can also elicit this reflex. It generally returns 1 to 3 days after the injury.

Autonomic dysfunction is worse with higher levels of injury. In cervical spinal cord injuries, the sympathetic outflow is diminished with a persistent parasympathetic output by the vagus nerve, resulting in bradycardia and hypotension. This autonomic dysfunction generally persists for months, and there is evidence to suggest that there is always some level of abnormality. Sympathetic activity can still be present and mediated by the spinal cord distal to the level of injury. Because of this sympathetic/parasympathetic imbalance, patients with complete spinal cord injury can have hypertensive crisis resulting from an overdistended bladder or colon.[2]

Because of this continuum of events after a spinal cord injury, the definition of spinal shock itself and the end point are variable. A recent article by Ditunno et al[3] describes spinal shock and the stages of reflexic recovery. This progression includes initial hyporeflexia (0 to 1 days), reflex return (1 to 3 days), early hyperreflexia (1 to 4 weeks), and late hyperreflexia (1 to 12 months).[3] In our institution, as in other level 1 trauma centers, we believe that spinal shock is at an end when the bulbocavernosus reflex returns.

References

1. Ko HY, Ditunno JF, Jr., Graziani V, et al. The pattern of reflex recovery during spinal shock. *Spinal Cord.* 1999;37:402-409.
2. Silver JR. Early autonomic dysreflexia. *Spinal Cord.* 2000;38:229-233.
3. Ditunno JF, Little JW, Tessler A, et al. Spinal shock revisited: a four-phase model. *Spinal Cord.* 2004;42:383-395.

QUESTION 24

I Have a 65-Year-Old Female Who Fell and Suffered a Central Cord Syndrome. What Is Her Prognosis and Are There Other Types of Incomplete Spinal Cord Syndromes?

Ahmad Nassr, MD and Joon Y. Lee, MD

Central cord syndrome is one of the incomplete spinal cord injuries with a relatively good prognosis (Table 24-1). This syndrome typically results in an asymmetric quadraparesis with weakness that is greater in the upper extremities than the lower extremities.[1] Sensation is involved to differing degrees, but patients frequently have sacral sparing. We generally see this type of incomplete spinal cord injury in elderly patients with pre-existing cervical spinal stenosis after a hyperextension injury (Figure 24-1). The spinal cord is pinched anteriorly between anterior osteophytes and posteriorly by buckling of the ligamentum flavum. This results in an injury to the grey and white matter in the central aspect of the spinal cord. The corticospinal tract is most severely involved, resulting in weakness of the upper extremities. Central cord syndrome responds favorably to decompression in the setting of moderate to severe cervical stenosis.

Other incomplete spinal cord injuries include anterior cord syndrome, Brown-Sequard syndrome, posterior cord syndrome, and conus medullaris syndrome. Cauda equina syndrome is sometimes included in the discussion of spinal cord injury, although it is not technically an injury to the cord but rather an injury to the roots below the level of the conus medullaris.

Anterior cord syndrome generally results from a hyperflexion injury. It is commonly confused with a complete spinal cord injury because it results in a complete loss of motor function, pain, and temperature sensation below the level of injury. Careful examination generally shows that some posterior column function remains intact, resulting in retention of proprioception, vibratory sense, and deep touch. This syndrome may also result

Table 24-1
Spinal Cord Syndromes

Syndrome	Findings
Anterior cord	• Damage from the ventral portion of the spinal cord o Interruption of the ascending spinothalamic tracts and descending motor tracts • Loss of pain and temperature sensation and motor control • Preservation of posterior column (proprioception/vibratory sensation) • Worst prognosis
Central cord	• Usually associated with cervical spondylosis and a hyperextension injury • Hands are usually more severely compromised • More significant injuries impair upper extremity motor function more than lower extremity motor function • Approximately 50% will regain ambulatory function
Posterior cord	• Disruption of the dorsal column tracts • Loss of proprioception and vibratory sensation • Extremely uncommon
Brown-Sequard	• Hemisection injury of the spinal cord • Ipsilateral loss of motor control • Contralateral loss of pain and temperature sensation below the level of the lesion • Best prognosis

Figure 24-1. MRI of a patient with pre-existing spinal stenosis who suffered a fall, which resulted in central cord syndrome. The white arrow shows new signal changes to the spinal cord, indicating injury.

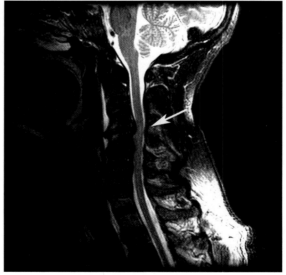

from an injury to the anterior spinal artery. Generally this injury has a poor prognosis for recovery.

Brown-Sequard syndrome may result from penetrating trauma such as a knife or bullet wound, herniated disk, or asymmetric rotational injuries, resulting in unilateral lamina, pedicle fractures, or facet injury. Patients present with the loss of motor function on the ipsilateral side of the injury and contralateral loss of pain and temperature sensation. This injury has the most favorable functional recovery of all the incomplete spinal cord injuries.

Posterior cord syndrome generally results from a hyperextension injury that causes disruption of the posterior columns with a resultant loss of deep touch, proprioception, and vibratory sensation. This form of incomplete injury is very rare.

Reference

1. Harrop JS, Sharan A, Ratliff J. Central cord injury: pathophysiology, management, and outcomes. *Spine.* 2006;6:S198-206.

25

I HAVE 57-YEAR-OLD MALE INVOLVED IN A HIGH SPEED MOTOR VEHICLE ACCIDENT. HE IS A C7 ASIA A WHO WENT TO THE EMERGENCY ROOM 12 HOURS AFTER HIS ACCIDENT. SHOULD I GIVE HIM INTRAVENOUS STEROIDS?

Ahmad Nassr, MD and Joon Y. Lee, MD

The use of steroids for spinal cord injury has been a recent topic of debate among spine surgeons. In our institution, we still use methylprednisolone if patients with spinal cord injuries are seen within 8 hours of their injury. This rationale is based upon the National Acute Spinal Cord Injury Study (NASCIS) guidelines (30 mg/kg bolus over 15 min, then administration of 5.4 mg/kg/h for either 24 hours (if the patient is seen within 3 hours of injury) or 48 hours if the patient is seen within 3 to 8 hours of the injury).

In the current clinical scenario, the patient is outside of the 8-hour window, and we would not initiate the steroid protocol. We still use steroids on a case-by-case basis even outside of this window of time, especially in the setting of incomplete spinal cord injuries. Recently, the results of the NASCIS studies have come under scrutiny. There is concern about the reproducibility of the study, and most spine surgeons disagree about the validity of the findings.[1-3] In a recent review of the literature, Hugenholtz et al found insufficient evidence to suggest the routine use of methylprednisolone as treatment for spinal cord injuries.[4]

The use of high-dose steroids has been theorized to increase the risk of medical complications and in recent studies has been related to an increased incidence of pulmonary complications. These issues should not be taken lightly because they can lead to life-threatening situations. These factors have brought about a recent push to abandon steroid use as the standard of care for acute spinal cord injury.

References

1. Coleman WP, Benzel D, Cahill DW, et al. A critical appraisal of the reporting of the National Acute Spinal Cord Injury Studies (II and III) of methylprednisolone in acute spinal cord injury. *J Spinal Disord.* 2000;13:185-199.
2. Eck JC, Nachtigall D, Humphreys SC, et al. Questionnaire survey of spine surgeons on the use of methylprednisolone for acute spinal cord injury. *Spine.* 2006;31:E250-253.
3. Galandiuk S, Raque G, Appel S, et al. The two-edged sword of large-dose steroids for spinal cord trauma. *Ann Surg.* 1993;218:419-425; discussion 25-27.
4. Hugenholtz H, Cass DE, Dvorak MF, et al. High-dose methylprednisolone for acute closed spinal cord injury—only a treatment option. *Can J Neurol Sci.* 2002;29:227-235.

SECTION VIII

DEGENERATIVE

I HAVE A 34-YEAR-OLD PATIENT WHO HAS HAD BACK PAIN AND SOME BUTTOCK PAIN FOR 2 WEEKS. WHEN SHOULD I GET AN MRI?

Brian Kwon, MD

In a young healthy patient, low back pain (LBP) for 2 weeks is considered acute (up to 6 weeks of duration). Buttock pain is noteworthy; however, facet joint and sacroiliac joint (SIJ) pain may mimic and contribute to buttock pain. Injection studies of the SIJ and facet joints at L4-5 and L5-S1 have found a region that localizes to the buttock in and around the posterior-superior iliac spine. It is a rather nonspecific location that does not offer any clues about the source of pain. His buttock pain is unlikely to represent true radiculopathy.

In this patient, an MRI is not indicated unless there is suspicion for more serious underlying disease. Infection, tumors, or trauma can be ruled out by a good history. A history of fevers, night pain/sweats, intravenous drug abuse, falls or high-energy blunt trauma (motor vehicle accident [MVA]), and nonmechanical pain (rest pain, pain not associated with activity) should alert you to these diagnoses.

The American College of Radiology has published appropriateness criteria for imaging in acute LBP.[1] Without a history of radiculopathy—typically pain radiating distal to the knee—an MRI and even x-rays score 2 out of 9 for appropriateness (9 being most appropriate). Acute diagnostic imaging of mechanical back pain is unlikely to alter management decisions and more importantly will create unnecessary procedures, further diagnostic workup, and excessive costs.

If you suspect cauda equina syndrome (CES: saddle anesthesia, bladder/bowel incontinence/retention, lower extremity pain/weakness) your patient should have an MRI as soon as possible. Once the diagnosis is confirmed, there is little role for nonsurgical treatment.

Remember the high incidence of abnormal MRI studies in asymptomatic individuals. Boden et al studied MRI findings in asymptomatic individuals in three different age categories. The authors looked at four common findings: disc herniation, disc bulges, disc degeneration, and spinal stenosis. They found that stenosis, disc bulges, and particularly disc degeneration increased in frequency with increasing age. In this patient's age group, disc bulges were noted in 55% of individuals.[2] Degenerative discs on MRI may be ubiquitous findings and should not be the factor on which you make any treatment decisions.

A prospective, randomized trial studied the prognostic role of early MRI in patients with acute LBP. Patients with acute (less than 2 weeks) LBP were all imaged with MRI. Patients were randomized to an early disclosure and a nondisclosure group. Those given the results of their MRI early did not demonstrate a difference in recovery compared to the group who did not receive their imaging results during a 6-week study period. In fact, the early-informed patients had a lesser sense of overall well-being.[3]

The natural history for acute, uncomplicated LBP is benign and carries an excellent prognosis. Assure your patient. If in 6 to 12 weeks the patient returns with persistent LBP, an MRI is appropriate as that time frame falls outside the routine recovery period. MRI has been shown to detect abnormalities (such as neoplasms) more often in this population.[4] Overall, MRI in acute LBP has been shown to have modest clinical benefit and may lead to increased costs of care and unnecessary concern by patients and physicians.

References

1. Anderson RE, Drayer BP, Braffman B, et al. Acute low back pain—radiculopathy, American College of Radiology, ACR Appropriateness Criteria. *Radiology.* 2000;215 Suppl:479-485.
2. Boden SD, Davis DO, Dina TS, Patronas NJ, Weisel SW. Abnormal magnetic resonance scans of the lumbar spine in asymptomatic individuals: a prospective investigation. *JBJS Am.* 1990;72(8):1178-1184.
3. Modic MT, Obuchowski NA, Ross JS, Brant-Zawadzki MN, Groof PN, Benzel EC. Acute low back pain and radiculopathy: MR imaging findings and their prognostic role and effect on outcome. *Radiology.* 2005;237(2): 597-604.
4. McNally EG, Wilson DJ, Ostlere SJ. Limited magnetic resonance imaging in low back pain instead of plain radiographs: experience with first 1000 cases. *Clin Radiol.* 2005; 56(1): 922-925.

I Have a 42-Year-Old Male With a Symptomatic Lumbar Disc Herniation That Has Been Present for 6 Weeks. What Roles Do Therapy and Epidural Injections Have?

Brian Kwon, MD

The first thing to remember is the favorable natural history of symptomatic lumbar disc herniations (LDH). Numerous authors have shown that the natural history of LDH treated with or without surgery is similar after as little as 2 years of follow-up. These studies also demonstrate that short-term results (less than 2 years) favor surgical intervention. Although surgery does not alter the long-term history, it certainly provides patients with LDH an accelerated return to work, household activities, and pain relief.

Initial treatment of LDH should be conservative for 6 weeks unless progressive neurological deficit or cauda equina syndrome (CES) is present. There are many therapies that can be instituted but their efficacy has not been supported with high-quality studies. Bed rest may be unavoidable, particularly when pain is acute and severe. There are no studies to support the use of prolonged bed rest for acute sciatica. Given the potential complications of recumbency, recommendations for inactivity and long-term bed rest should be avoided and kept to less than 48 hours. Traction for sciatica can be of some benefit but has not been shown to lead to any long-term pain relief or decreased rates of surgery. A Cochrane review in 2005 stated that traction is probably not effective compared to other placebo treatments for decreasing pain, disability, and lost time from work.[1]

Injections are controversial in the management of LDH. Their use has good rationale because the pain from LDH herniations is mediated through inflammatory mechanisms. A meta-analysis of 4 randomized trials found epidural steroid injections (ESI) more beneficial (odds ratio of 2.2) for control of acute sciatic pain, particularly at short follow-up periods. Again, there were no differences in long-term pain relief.[2] In a randomized controlled trial of 100 patients with symptomatic LDH treated with ESI or surgical discectomy, Buttermann[3] found that 92 to 96% of patients treated with discectomy reported a successful outcome, whereas only 42 to 56% of patients in the ESI group felt their treatment was effective. Additionally, there were 27 patients who crossed over from the ESI to the surgical group. ESI offered good pain relief in up to 50% of patients and did not negatively impact results of future surgery. The author concluded that ESI is less effective overall compared to surgery for the treatment of pain due to LDH.[3]

There has been recent interest in fluoroscopically guided transforaminal epidural steroid injections (TFESI) for the treatment of symptomatic LDH. Several studies have shown that TFESI can offer good pain relief and reduce the need for surgery.[4] Vad et al reported on a series of 48 nonrandomized patients receiving TFESI or a saline trigger point injection (TPI). They found successful results (patient reported, Roland-Morris, more than 50% pain relief on VAS, lumbar flexibility) in 84% of patients who received TFESI compared to 48% in the TPI group. The follow-up period was 1.4 years, and patients received an average of 1.7 injections.[5] Riew et al published a study of 55 patients with LDH who were deemed candidates for surgical discectomy after a minimum of 6 weeks of conservative care. All patients received TFESI but were randomized to groups with or without steroids in the injection. In the steroid group, 71% elected not to proceed with surgery compared to 33% in the group that did not receive steroids. The average follow-up was 23 months, and the patients received an average of 1.6 injections.[6] A follow-up study reported 80% of the patient who avoided surgery continued to do so 5 years later.[7]

The Spine Patient Outcomes Research Trial (SPORT) was designed to provide level I evidence comparing surgical to nonsurgical treatment of symptomatic LDH; 501 patients were randomized to operative and nonoperative groups. The nonsurgical group underwent care that consisted of education/counseling (93%), medications (60%), injections (56%), and active therapy (44%). After 2 years, there were notable differences in favor of surgical intervention, but none were statistically significant. At all time points prior to the 2-year follow-up, surgical patients noted an improved visual analog scale (VAS) leg pain score and an increased activity level and return to work. There was a high rate of crossover (in both directions), which precluded any firm conclusion regarding the superiority of one treatment over the other.[8]

These data suggest that for a symptomatic LDH lasting longer than 6 weeks, therapy has no specific role for treatment but injections may. The superiority of interlaminar ESI versus TFESI has not been rigorously examined. There is a suggestion that TFESI may be more effective and may change the natural history of symptomatic LDH if surgery is considered the main endpoint. However, whether the patients who avoid surgery consider their own treatment a success has not been examined.

References

1. Clarke JA, van Tulder MW, Blomberg SE, de Vet HC, van der Heijden GJ, Bronfort G. Traction for low back pain with or without sciatica. *Cochrane Database Syst Rev.* 2005;4:CD003010.
2. Vroomen PC, de Krom MC, Slofstra PD, Knottnerus JA. Conservative treatment of sciatica: a systematic review. *Spinal Disord.* 2000;13:463-469.
3. Buttermann GR. Treatment of lumbar disc herniation: epidural steroid injection compared with discectomy: a prospective, randomized study. *J Bone Joint Surg Am.* 2004;86:670-679.
4. DePalma MJ, Bhargava A, Slipman CW. A critical appraisal of the evidence for selective nerve root injection in the treatment of lumbosacral radiculopathy. *Arch Phys Med Rehabil.* 2005;86(7):1477-1483.

5. Vad VB, Bhat AL, Lutz GE, Cammisa F. Transforaminal epidural steroid injections in lumbosacral radiculopathy: a prospective randomized study. *Spine.* 2002;27:11-16.

6. Riew KD, Yin Y, Gilula L, et al. The effect of nerve-root injections on the need for operative treatment of lumbar radicular pain: a prospective, randomized, controlled, double-blind study. *J Bone Joint Surg Am.* 2000;82:1589-1593.

7. Riew KD, Park JB, Cho YS, et al. Nerve root blocks in the treatment of lumbar radicular pain: a minimum five-year follow-up. *J Bone Joint Surg Am.* 2006;88(8):1722-1725.

8. Weinstein JN, Lurie JD, Tosteson TD, et al. Surgical vs nonoperative treatment for lumbar disk herniation: the Spine Patient Outcomes Research Trial (SPORT) observational cohort. *JAMA.* 2006;296(20):2451-2459.

28

I Have a 67-Year-Old Female With a T7 Compression Fracture. Are There Any Findings That Can Help Me to Differentiate a Pathological Compression Fracture From an Osteoporotic Fracture?

Brian Kwon, MD

Benign osteoporotic compression fractures are common in elderly individuals. Unfortunately, metastatic disease is also seen in the same population. Before you even look at the magnetic resonance imaging (MRI) scan, take into consideration the patient's history. Has she had any recent trauma such as low-energy falls? Does she have a prior history of cancer? Has she complained recently about pain at rest or at night? Does she have a recent history of fevers or weight loss? If there are no differentiating clues in her history, then the MRI may provide you with some invaluable information.

Link et al suggested compression fractures above T7 with paraspinal soft tissue masses are very likely to be malignant.[1] Additionally, Baur et al noted that the fluid sign—bone marrow edema adjacent to an endplate, signal intensity isointense to cerebral spinal fluid (CSF)—is suggestive of a benign compression fracture.[2]

Jung and colleagues[3] retrospectively reviewed MRI findings of 27 patients with pathologic compression fractures and 55 with benign osteoporotic compression fractures. A radiologist blinded to the diagnosis read all films. The mean age was 57 years for the metastatic group and 69 years for the osteoporotic group. Men constituted 70% of the metastatic group, but women were 73% of the osteoporotic group. They found specific MRI characteristics that were significantly different:

- Osteoporotic lesions
    - A low signal intensity band on T1- and T2-weighted images

- o Spared, normal bone marrow signal intensity
- o Retropulsion of the posterior cortex into the canal
- o Multiple compression fractures
- • Metastatic lesions
  - o Convex posterior vertebral body cortex
  - o Involvement of pedicles and posterior elements
  - o Epidural mass that may encase the neural elements
  - o A focal paraspinal mass
  - o Other spinal metastatic lesions

Baur et al used diffusion-weighted MRIs to differentiate between osteoporotic and malignant compression fractures. Diffusion weighting reflects the mobility of water molecules in interstitial tissue that will display signal attenuation. This allows for better tissue characterization. They found that benign osteoporotic compression fractures showed hypointense to isointense signal characteristics compared to adjacent vertebral bodies when diffusion weighting was applied. Conversely, malignant compression fractures became hyperintense after diffusion weighting. Differences in signal characteristics on fast spin echo (FSE) or short tau inversion-recovery (STIR) sequences were minimal between the two conditions.[4]

References

1. Link TM, Guglielmi G, van Kuijk C, Adams JE. Radiologic assessment of osteoporotic vertebral fractures: diagnostic and prognostic implications. *Eur Radiol.* 2005;15:1521-1532.
2. Baur A, Stabler A, Arbogast S, Duerr HR, Bartl R, Reiser M. Acute osteoporotic and neoplastic vertebral compression fractures: fluid sign at MR imaging. *Radiology.* 2002;225(3):730-735.
3. Jung HS, Jee WH, McCauley TR, Ha KY, Choi KH. Discrimination of metastatic from acute osteoporotic compression spinal fractures with MR imaging. *Radiographics.* 2003;23(1):179-187.
4. Baur A, Stabler A, Bruning R, et al. Diffusion-weighted MR imaging of bone marrow: differentiation of benign versus pathologic compression fractures. *Radiology.* 1998;207(2):349-356.

I HAVE A 72-YEAR-OLD FEMALE WITH A SYMPTOMATIC T12 VERTEBRAL COMPRESSION FRACTURE THAT HAS FAILED A COURSE OF BRACING. HOW DO I DECIDE WHETHER SHE SHOULD UNDERGO A KYPHOPLASTY OR A VERTEBROPLASTY?

Brian Kwon, MD

Osteoporotic vertebral compression fractures (OVCF) affect up to 25% of postmenopausal women. The frequency reported in the United States is 700,000 per year, which is more than double the annual incidence of hip fractures. A single OVCF increases the risk of a subsequent OCVF by five times. Although most OVCF recover without incident in 6 to 12 weeks, up to 30% of patients who seek care do not have adequate pain relief.[1]

Chronic pain from OVCF leads to increased morbidity from prolonged use of medications and bed rest, poor appetite and nutrition, decreased pulmonary function, and overall poor quality of life. There is also some suggestion that mortality may be increased. The prolonged course of conservative management—bed rest, medication, and bracing—has led to the development of percutaneous cement injection into the fractured vertebrae.

Kyphoplasty (KP) involves inflating a balloon in the vertebral body prior to injection of cement (Figure 29-1). Vertebroplasty (VP) involves cement placement, without a balloon, into the fractured vertebral body. Once your patient has failed a 6-week course of conservative treatment, she may want to consider KP or VP. The superiority of one procedure over the other has not been determined in high-quality level I studies.

Taylor et al[2] performed a literature review and meta-analysis on VP and KP. They analyzed two nonrandomized controlled studies and 57 case series on VP. For KP, they

Figure 29-1. Schematic of the inflatable balloon used in kyphoplasty prior to cement injection. The balloon allows for vertebral height restoration and low-pressure cement injection.

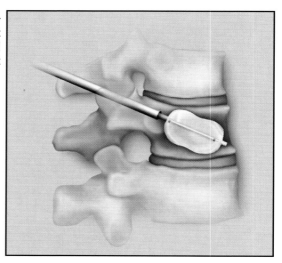

examined 4 nonrandomized comparative studies and 13 case series. In the comparative studies (VP or KP versus medical care), pain relief was significantly better after both VP and KP. Pain relief was similar in the one study comparing VP and KP, albeit with a short 4.5-month follow-up.[3] Similar results were seen when functional outcomes were measured: VP and KP performed better than medical care. Follow-up times and outcomes measurements were not standardized, so no direct comparisons could be made. Height restoration and kyphosis correction were not significantly different between VP and KP. The authors examined procedural safety and found significant differences in complications between the two procedures. The pooled data showed that the rate of cement leakage (40%, of which 3% were symptomatic) and pulmonary embolism in the VP group were significantly higher. No differences in rates of subsequent fractures were noted.

Hulme and colleagues reported similar outcomes for pain relief and function. From their pooled data, they found both KP and VP changed alignment by an average of 6.6 degreees. They also showed 34% of KP and 39% of VP procedures showed no height restoration or change in kyphosis. Cement leakage and complications were higher in the VP group than the KP group.[4]

In the end, there is only class III evidence that VP and KP are effective and have positive outcomes. There are no published, randomized controlled trials comparing the efficacy and safety of KP and VP. Based on expert opinion only, if the patient is able to undergo KP, then this may be a better alternative for correction of sagittal height and pain relief. On the other hand, if the patient cannot tolerate a general anesthesia, VP may be preferred. There are no firm recommendations beyond opinion and comfort level of the treating physician.

References

1. Kim DH, Vaccaro AR. Osteoporotic compression fractures of the spine: current options and considerations for treatment. *Spine.* 2006;6(5):479-487.
2. Taylor RS, Taylor RJ, Fritzell P. Balloon kyphoplasty and vertebroplasty for vertebral compression fractures: a comparative systematic review of efficacy and safety. *Spine.* 2006;31(23):2747-2755.
3. Fourney DR, Schomer DF, Nader R, et al. Percutaneous vertebroplasty and kyphoplasty for painful vertebral body fractures in cancer patients. *J Neurosurg.* 2003;98(1 Suppl):21-30.
4. Hulme PA, Krebs J, Ferguson SJ, Berlemann U. Vertebroplasty and kyphoplasty: a systematic review of 69 clinical studies. *Spine.* 2006;31(17):1983-2001.

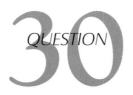

30

I Have a 34-Year-Old Male With Cervical Myelopathy and Multiple-Level Cervical Stenosis. I Am Concerned About Performing a Posterior Cervical Fusion on Such a Young Patient. Are There Any Alternatives That Would Treat His Myelopathy and Preserve His Neck Range of Motion?

Brian Kwon, MD

There are several ways to surgically treat cervical myelopathy. Anterior cervical corpectomy and discectomy with fusion is an option. Laminoplasty and laminectomy with fusion are the posterior options. Both anterior and posterior approaches have been shown to have similar outcomes in several retrospective studies. Laminectomy alone is no longer performed because late kyphosis and usually recurrent myelopathy can occur in up to 25% of patients.[1]

Laminoplasty is not typically done with concomitant fusion. There are two main techniques: open door and French door (Figures 30-1A, B, and C). The open door procedure involves an osteotomy of the cervical lamina combined with "hinging" the contralateral lamina. The French door technique hinges on both laminae that are divided in the middle. Both techniques allow for expansion of the cervical canal and decompression of the spinal cord (Figure 30-1B). Laminoplasty can address multiple levels of cervical stenosis even when the major pathological entity is anterior to the spinal cord. It does require lordotic or neutral alignment of the cervical spine. Wada et al[2] reported a retrospective minimum 10-year follow-up of 47 patients who underwent either anterior corpectomy and fusion or laminoplasty. There were similar rates of neurological recovery in both groups. Measured radiographically, cervical range of motion (ROM) in the corpectomy and fusion group decreased 49% and in the laminaplasty group by 29%; this difference was significant.[2] Seichi et al reported a minimum 10-year follow-up after laminoplasty using the French door technique. They found ROM decreased 75% (36 degrees to 8 degrees) and 54% had complete fusion. Laminoplasty was initially intended to preserve motion and avoid complications common to fusion. Long-term studies of laminoplasty show that radiographic ROM decreases but still provides more motion than anterior decompression and fusion.[3]

In this patient, laminoplasty will provide surgical decompression of his stenotic cervical canal, while allowing him to preserve ROM, which is essential in a young, active individual.

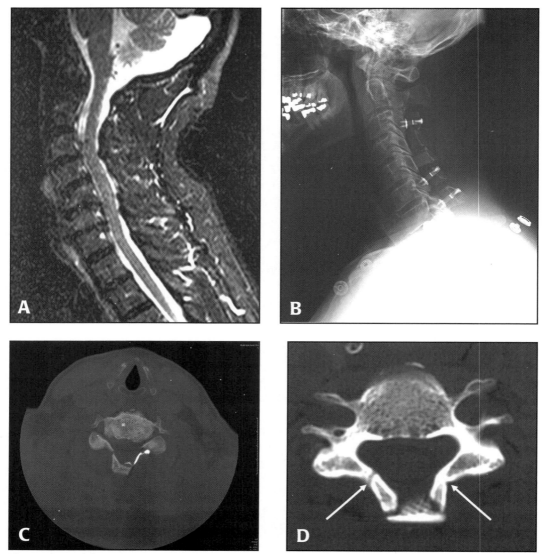

Figure 30-1. (A) Sagital cervical MRI demonstrating multiple-level spinal cord compression. (B) Lateral postoperative radiograph demonstrating bone graft and laminoplasty plate fixation. (C) Axial CT scan demonstrating the laminoplasty plate used to buttress open the lamina in the open door technique. (D) Axial CT scan image demonstrating a spinous process autograft used to wedge open the lamina in the French door technique.

References

1. Kaptain GJ, Simmons NE, Replogle RE, Pobereskin L. Incidence and outcome of kyphotic deformity following laminectomy for cervical spondylotic myelopathy. *J Neurosurg.* 2000;93(2 Suppl):199-204.
2. Wada E, Suzuki S, Kanazawa A, Matsuoka T, Miyamoto S, Yonenobu K. Subtotal corpectomy versus laminoplasty for multilevel cervical spondylotic myelopathy: a long-term follow-up study over 10 years. *Spine.* 2001;26(13):1443-1447.
3. Seichi A, Takeshita K, Ohishi I, et al. Long-term results of double-door laminoplasty for cervical stenotic myelopathy. *Spine.* 2001;26(5):479-487.

31

I HAVE A 29-YEAR-OLD MALE WITH RIGHT ARM PAIN DUE TO A C6 DISC HERNIATION. IS THERE A SURGICAL ALTERNATIVE TO AN ANTERIOR CERVICAL DISCECTOMY AND FUSION IN THIS PATIENT?

Brian Kwon, MD

There are several options for treating cervical radiculopathy involving anterior and posterior approaches. The anterior options include cervical discectomy and fusion or anterior cervical foraminotomy (ACF). Posterior cervical foraminotomy (PCF) is a common and well-described procedure for treating cervical radiculopathy.

PCF is a less invasive approach to treating cervical radiculopathy. It is best done on patients with unilateral, one- or two-level disease without significant spondylosis at other levels. It is particularly good when facet joint arthropathy and soft disc herniations are major causative factors of nerve root compression.

The major advantage of PCF is that there is no need for fusion. Resection of between 25% and 50% of the facet joint has been shown to provide adequate decompression of the nerve root. Greater than 50% resection may lead to instability and should be carefully observed after the operation. Additionally, complications unique to the anterior approach—esophageal injury, dysphagia, and vertebral artery injury—are avoided. The major disadvantages are the inability to address bilateral pathology and the belief that the posterior incision is more painful. With endoscopic techniques, postoperative neck pain may be minimized.

Results after PCF have been excellent in many long-term series. Patient-reported outcomes reveal 92% to 96% of patients have excellent and good outcomes. Complications are rare (2.2%). Most involve major blood loss and CSF leaks.[1]

Figure 31-1. Axial CT scan. The arrow represents the fifth cervical nerve root in the neuroforamen. The cylinder is the area of the uncinate to be resected. The star represents the vertebral artery.

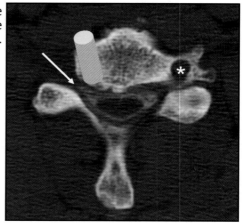

ACF uses the familiar Smith-Robinson approach and involves direct decompression of the nerve root in the foramen (Figure 31-1). The advantages of this procedure are that it (1) does not require fusion, as disc resection is minimal, (2) directly addresses anterior pathology, and (3) can be done microsurgically with minimal morbidity. It should be used for unilateral, one- or two-level pathology.[2] The approach starts at the antero-lateral aspect of the vertebral body and is directed at the neuroforamen. Using a high-speed burr, the uncus is resected back to the posterior annulus and posterior longitudinal ligament.

References

1. Epstein N. Posterior approaches in the management of cervical spondylosis and ossification of the posterior longitudinal ligament. *Surg Neurol.* 2002;58(3-4):194-207.
2. Bruneau M, Cornelius JF, George B. Microsurgical cervical nerve root decompression by anterolateral approach. *Neurosurgery.* 2006;58(1 Suppl):ONS108-113.

32

WHAT IS THE DIFFERENCE BETWEEN CERVICAL MYELOPATHY AND RADICULOPATHY?

Brian Kwon, MD

Simply said, myelopathy is a disease of the spinal cord, and radiculopathy is a disease of the nerve roots. Cervical myelopathy (CM) is commonly seen in older individuals (50s and 60s) and is common in Asian countries. The most frequent causes of CM are spondylosis, ossification of the posterior longitudinal ligament (OPLL), and disk herniations. The pathophysiology of CM is thought to be ischemia from spinal cord compression. The chronically ischemic spinal cord undergoes irreversible changes that lead to cord dysfunction and to symptoms of CM. Congenital cervical stenosis predisposes patients to CM, because narrower spinal canals are less tolerant of compression from osteophytes and discs.

The presentation of CM can be subtle. Bilateral hand numbness, motor weakness in the upper extremities (UE), and gait abnormalities are the most common symptoms. Patients will complain of changes in handwriting, fine finger movements, and ambulation. Bladder and bowel dysfunction can occur late in the disease. The natural history of CM is thought to progress in a stepwise fashion in a majority of patients. However, recent studies by Kadanka et al[1] have reported that although mild myelopathy may not progress significantly after 5 years, it should be followed because some progression can occur.

The diagnosis of CM is made with history, physical findings, and imaging studies. Typical findings include hyperreflexia, wide-based gait, and pathological reflexes such as a Hoffman's (Figure 32-1) or Babinski's sign (Figure 32-2). Imaging studies should include upright radiographs and magnetic resonance imaging (MRI). Radiographic studies can assess cervical alignment but also provide evidence of subluxation and instability. MRI is the test of choice to assess for spinal cord compression. Many authors argue about how to define true canal compromise: absolute (less than 8 mm) and relative (Torg ratio less than 0.8) values have been reported. Deformation of the spinal cord has also been studied.

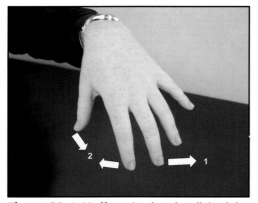

Figure 32-1. Hoffman's sign is elicited by hyperextension of the distal interphalangeal joint of the middle finger (stage I) and observing a reflexic contraction of the thumb and index finger (stage II).

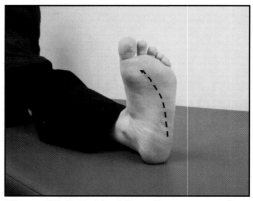

Figure 32-2. Babinski's reflex occurs when the great toe flexes toward the top of the foot and the other toes fan out after the sole of the foot has been firmly stroked.

Figure 32-3. Cervical nerve root compression. The arrow represents posterolateral vertebral osteophytes. The star represents osteophytes from the facet joint contributing to the narrowing of the neural foramen.

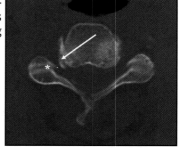

Cord signal changes on T2- and T1-weighted sequences are thought to have prognostic implications as well.

Treatment is primarily surgical and involves decompression from anterior or posterior approaches with or without fusion. The timing of surgery in CM has been debated. Many surgeons would agree that once the patient becomes symptomatic and has documented cord compression surgical intervention is warranted.

Cervical radiculopathy (CR) results from cervical nerve root compression, which leads to upper extremity pain and sometimes weakness. CR is seen in a wide variety of ages, but the average age is younger than that of CM. Nerve root compression can be caused by disc herniation and osteophytes from the facet joint, uncovertebral joint, and annulus (Figure 32-3). Patients complain of arm pain more than neck pain. Radiculopathy has not been strongly associated with neck pain alone. The location is typically dermatomal and may course past the shoulder to the elbow and wrist. Motor weakness and reflex changes can be seen as well also in a segmental pattern. Shoulder pathology (rotator cuff disease, impingement) and peripheral neuropathies (carpal tunnel, cubital tunnel) can often overlap and should be looked for and ruled out.

Imaging studies in CR should include x-rays, but the study of choice is MRI. Spinal cord compression should be assessed, but the cardinal finding is typically foraminal stenosis. There has been no study directly correlating amount of foraminal stenosis and symptoms before or after surgery.[2] Also given the size of the foramen and MRI slices, true stenosis can be under- or overestimated. Computed tomography after myelography can yield information that is not well imaged on MRI.

The natural history of CR overall is very favorable. Up to 75% of patients will have good resolution of their pain within 6 to 12 weeks. Medications, therapy, and injections have been shown to have variable short-term results and some long-term benefit. Persistent radicular pain for longer than 6 weeks and failure of conservative therapy is a good indication for surgical intervention. Progressive motor loss and/or myelopathy may preclude conservative care. Surgical options include anterior and posterior procedures. The majority of patients with CR have a favorable prognosis with 85 to 92% having good to excellent results (pain relief and motor recovery) after surgical intervention.

References

1. Kadanka Z, Mares M, Bednarik J, et al. Approaches to spondylotic cervical myelopathy: conservative versus surgical results in a 3-year follow-up study. *Spine.* 2002;27(20):2205-2210.
2. Albert TJ, Smith MD, Bressler E, Johnson LJ. An in vivo analysis of the dimensional changes of the neuroforamen after anterior cervical diskectomy and fusion: a radiologic investigation. *J Spinal Disord.* 1997;10(3):229-233.

I Have a 29-Year-Old Male With a Large Central Disc Herniation at L4-5. He States That He Has Had Difficulty With Urination. How Do I Make Sure He Does Not Have Cauda Equina Syndrome?

Brian Kwon, MD

Cauda equina syndrome (CES) classically presents as low back pain, bilateral or unilateral sciatica, and bladder or bowel retention/incontinence due to neural compression in the lumbar spine. We know that the components of CES that involve pain are recoverable and certainly not harmful per se. It is the urogenital symptoms that are most concerning because of their morbidity and irreversibility.

Urinary retention is a common early sign heralding CES. Retention typically happens well before presentation and is often noted as a subjective complaint rather than objective finding. At 29 years old, your patient is unlikely to have other causes of urinary retention outside of CES. Typical causes can be categorized into obstructive, neurogenic, pharmacologic, and psychiatric etiologies. The classic obstructive causes are prostate enlargement, urethral strictures, and kidney stones. In older men, prostate problems should be inquired about and early evaluation by an urologist is needed. A history of urethritis and urethral strictures, which in your patient would most likely be due to infections from sexually transmitted diseases, may also be a cause of urinary retention. Renal stones are an obstructive cause of urinary retention. In this case, flank pain may be confused with low back pain. Pharmacologic causes of retention include heroin and demerol use. To treat pain, these drugs may have been initiated by the patient or prescribed by his physician. Prostate disease, urethritis, and stones can be ruled out with physical examination, blood and urine tests, and imaging modalities. Again, consultation with a urologist might be helpful if there is any suspicion of these diagnoses.

Figure 33-1. Schematic of a large, central lumbar disc herniation causing severe compression of the cauda equina.

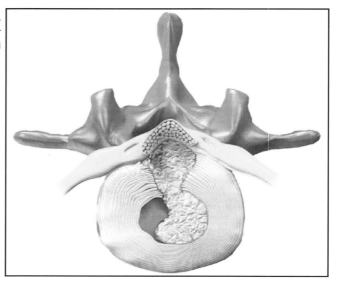

Once the diagnosis of CES is made, treatment is surgical decompression (Figure 33-1). Some authors recommend a complete laminectomy prior to discectomy to minimize manipulation of already compromised neural structures.[1] Ahn et al[2] performed a meta-analysis of outcomes following surgical management of CES. Their cardinal finding was that patients operated on within 24 hours and between 24 and 48 hours of onset of CES had equivalent outcomes. There were significant differences in outcomes when patients were operated on after 48 hours of CES symptoms. Patients operated on beyond 48 hours were at 2.5 times the risk of a persistent urinary deficit, 9.1 times the risk of a persistent motor deficit, 9.1 times the risk of continuing rectal dysfunction, and 3.5 times the risk of a sensory deficit. Other risk factors for poor outcomes were chronic low back pain, rectal dysfunction, and urinary incontinence at presentation.

The sine qua non of CES is cauda equina compression. It is typically caused by a large disc herniation or a smaller herniation combined with spinal stenosis. In the analysis by Ahn et al, only 38% were due to disk herniations at L4-L5 or L5-S1.[2] Hernations at other levels should not be underestimated. Overall outcomes can be good. Of patients who had surgery beyond 48 hours, 83% reported pain relief, 75% motor recovery, 73% recovery of urinary continence, 67% sexual function, 64% rectal function, and 56% sensory restoration.[2]

References

1. Shapiro S. Medical realities of cauda equina syndrome secondary to lumbar disc herniation. *Spine.* 2000;25(3):348-351.
2. Ahn UM, Ahn NU, Buchowski JM, Garrett ES, Sieber AN, Kostuik JP. Cauda equina syndrome secondary to lumbar disc herniation: a meta-analysis of surgical outcomes. *Spine.* 2000;25(12):1515-1522.

SECTION IX

PEDIATRICS

34

I HAVE A 12-YEAR-OLD MALE WITH A 3-MONTH HISTORY OF BACK PAIN THAT DOES NOT APPEAR TO BE RESOLVING. HOW SHOULD I WORK UP BACK PAIN IN AN ADOLESCENT?

Shay Bess, MD

Approximately 36% of adolescents report at least one episode of substantial back pain, and approximately 7% seek medical attention for the condition.[1] In contradistinction to adults, back pain in the pediatric population commonly has a specific organic etiology. Pain that radiates into the lower extremities, the presence of neurological symptoms including sensory or motor deficits, and/or symptoms present for longer than 4 weeks are uncommon in adolescents and should motivate a thorough evaluation. The most common etiologies of adolescent back pain include trauma, disc herniation, tumor, infection, spondylolysis/spondylolisthesis, and Scheuermann's kyphosis. Some key elements of the history as noted by the patient or, more often, by the parents, as well as unique aspects of the physical examination and diagnostic imaging can help elucidate the etiology of the patient's symptoms.

Apophyseal Ring Fracture (Figures 34-1)

- *Background.* Apophyseal ring fractures occur between the vertebral and cartilaginous endplates and are often associated with a discrete hyperflexion event or with repetitive microtrauma as may occur in athletes.

- *Pain.* Often acute onset with history of a discrete event. Pain onset may be insidious if associated with microtrauma from vigorous activities. Pain is often localized and may radiate into the buttocks but rarely radiates below the knees. Symptoms are exacerbated by lumbar flexion and Valsalva maneuvers.

Figure 34-1. Apophyseal ring fractures occur between the vertebral and cartilaginous endplates in the immature spine. Note the associated annulus disruption and nucleus pulposis herniation, often exacerbating the patient's back and leg pain.

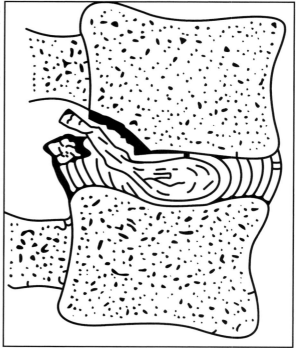

- *Additional Symptoms.* Neurological symptoms are not common but may be present if there is a large, posteriorly displaced bony fragment causing neural compression.

- *Physical Examination.* Regional tenderness may be present over the affected area. Straight leg raise is often positive. Weakness and numbness are less common.

- *Diagnostic Imaging.* Plain films may show a fragment posterior to the vertebral body at the disc space. Computed tomography (CT) is the imaging modality of choice and will show a posterior displaced cortical fragment at the endplate. The addition of myelography to the CT scan will help delineate if there is associated neural compression; however, this is a much more invasive procedure and may be poorly tolerated. Magnetic resonant imaging (MRI) will demonstrate if there is associated neural compression but often will not clearly differentiate cortical bone displacement from herniated disc material.

Disc Herniation

- *Background.* Lumbar disc herniation (LDH) is uncommon in the adolescent population and, unlike adults, is often a result of a traumatic event rather than a degenerative process. Up to 50% of LDH in adolescents involve a discrete traumatic event. Other risk factors include repetitive microtrauma due to strenuous activity.

- *Pain.* May be acute or insidious onset depending if there is a history of trauma. Pain often radiates into buttocks, posterior thigh, and the foot (sciatica). Coughing, sneezing, and other Valsalva maneuvers that increase intra-abdominal pressure exacerbate pain.

- *Additional Symptoms.* Numbness and weakness. May also report abnormal posture and gait when their "back goes out." Bowel and bladder symptoms are uncommon and can have a multitude of etiologies; however, if present, cauda equina syndrome must be ruled out with a thorough physical examination including perineal sensory and rectal exam.

- *Physical Examination.* Straight leg raise is positive in approximately 85% of patients. Neurological symptoms (weakness, numbness, and/or hyporeflexia) are less common, present in approximately 40% of patients. Other findings include listing posture and gait.

- *Diagnostic Imaging.* Plain films are reportedly normal in 50% of adolescents with LDH. A nonstructural scoliosis (sciatic scoliosis) is the most common finding on plain films. MRI is the imaging modality of choice. MRI will often demonstrate a large fragment because the herniated fragment is usually due to trauma, not degeneration, and is well hydrated.

Tumor

- *Background.* Primary spine tumors are uncommon, especially in the pediatric population. Most neoplasms that affect the adolescent spine are benign. Osteoid osteoma, osteoblastoma, and aneurysmal bone cyst are the most common. Eosinophilic granuloma most often affects younger children, not adolescents. Leukemia is the most common pediatric malignant neoplasm; however, it most often affects children younger than 10. Osteosarcoma and Ewing's sarcoma are rarely seen in the spine. Spinal metastasis is also uncommon the pediatric population. Neuroblastoma and rhabdomyosarcoma are the most common pediatric neoplasms that skeletally metastasize.

- *Pain.* Insidious onset, often progressive. Pain may radiate below the knees into lower extremities if there is associated neural compression by tumor or pathologic fracture. Pain that is worse at night, not relieved by rest, or when supine is concerning for malignancy. Pain that may be well relieved by NSAIDs is classically found in osteoid osteoma.

- *Additional Symptoms.* Malaise, weight loss, painful scoliosis that is not structural, and torticollis. Fevers are less common than in appendicular lesions (Ewing's sarcoma, metastatic disease). Neurological deficits may be present in up to 70% of pediatric patients with a malignant neoplasm.

- *Physical Examination.* Many patients will have local spinal tenderness; however, a palpable mass is less common than in the appendicular skeleton. Painful, nonstructural scoliosis with asymmetric forward bending is common. Neurological deficits are more common in malignant than benign lesions.

- *Diagnostic Imaging.* Plain film radiographs may demonstrate lytic, blastic, or mixed lesions. Vertebra plana may be demonstrated in eosinophilic granuloma or severe pathologic fracture. MRI is the modality of choice for initial evaluation and will demonstrate regions of signal change. CT can then be used to further define bony destruction in the regions delineated on the MRI. CT combined with technetium bone scan will help delineate lesions that are subtle on plain films (osteoid osteoma). Skeletal survey, bone scan, and CT of the chest, abdomen, and pelvis are most often indicated to rule out additional lesions and/or metastasis.

Infection

- *Background.* Pediatric vertebral osteomyelitis and discitis are a progressive infectious processes of hematologic etiology that initially affect the vertebral body and traverse the vertebral endplate to the adjacent disc. Staphylococcus aureus is reportedly the most common isolate.

- *Pain.* Insidious onset; symptoms are often progressive. Pain and tenderness is often well located in the back and may radiate into the buttock and lower extremities if there is associated neural compression by epidural abscess or nerve root irritation by an inflammatory process. Infection involving T8-L1 may cause abdominal pain.

- *Additional Symptoms.* Recent fevers, malaise, otitis media, pharyngitis, or flu/cold symptoms. Patients with epidural abscess are often not febrile; however, vertebral osteomyelitis/discitis is often preceded by bacterial or viral infection.[2]

- *Physical Examination.* Regional tenderness with local muscle spasm and loss of lumbar lordosis. Straight leg test is often positive. Patients with neural compression from an epidural abscess may demonstrate weakness, numbness, and hyporeflexia.

- *Diagnostic Imaging.* Radiographic changes are usually not evident before 3 weeks. Subsequent changes include loss of disc height and endplate erosions and sclerosis. MRI is the imaging modality of choice and will demonstrate the extent of the infection and the presence of an epidural abscess. Technetium bone scans will usually show increased uptake in the vertebral endplates and may also show additional skeletal lesions, especially in the appendicular skeleton.

- *Additional tests.* Complete blood count (CBC) with differential, erythrocyte sedimentation rate (ESR), and C-reactive protein (CRP) should be obtained in all patients with suspected osteomyelitis/discitis. ESR is the most sensitive laboratory test, because approximately 90% of patients will have elevated ESR. Conversely, as few as 10% will have an abnormal white blood cell count. Biopsy specimens and blood cultures will help direct antibiotic dosing if positive; however, Wenger et al reported that only 67% of biopsy specimens and 41% of blood cultures were positive in pediatric patients with suspected bacterial spine infections.[3]

Spondylolysis/Spondylolisthesis

- *Background.* Common cause of adolescent back pain. Reported prevalence is 4.4% in children. High incidence (47%) in adolescent athletes complaining of back pain. Also has a high incidence (50%) in association with Scheuermann's kyphosis. This condition is rarely symptomatic prior to the adolescent growth spurt.

- *Pain.* Often has an insidious onset; however, patients may have a history of an acute hyperextension event or may participate in activities requiring hyperextension (swimming, gymnastics, football, wrestling). Pain may radiate into buttocks and posterior thighs. Symptoms are exacerbated by flexion/extension activities and may prohibit participation in athletics. Symptoms are usually relieved by rest.

- *Additional Symptoms.* Low back stiffness with dramatically reduced lumbar flexion and stiff, shortened gait.

- *Physical Examination.* Hamstring tightness. Abnormal gait with short stride length. Reduced lumbar flexion may be dramatic. Large vertebral slippage may be associated with a palpable step-off (the spinous process of the affected vertebra is palpable because of posterior displacement through the pars defect). Buttocks may have a heart-shaped/vertical appearance and the frontal view of the patient may demonstrate transverse abdominal creases due to vertical sacral alignment. May also have abdominal protrusion due to compensatory lumbar hyperlordosis.

- *Diagnostic Imaging.* Upright AP, lateral, and flexion/extension radiographs will often demonstrate a bilateral pars defect and associated vertebral slip. Oblique radiographs may help delineate a pars abnormality (defect or elongation). Up to 20% of cases may have a unilateral pars defect and may require bone scan, single-photon emission computed tomography (SPECT), or CT to define the lesion. The pars defect may be difficult to visualize on CT axial images but is more readily seen on the sagittal reconstructions.

Scheuermann Kyphosis[4]

- *Background.* Estimated prevalence 0.4% to 8%. Primarily affects adolescents at puberty, with an equal male-female distribution. Must be differentiated from postural roundback or postural kyphosis.

- *Pain.* Insidious. Symptoms are often localized to the apex of the kyphosis. Pain is exacerbated by prolonged sitting or standing and by activities that require "good posture" (violin, piano playing, etc).

- *Additional Symptoms.* Family and teachers often note "poor posture."

- *Physical Examination.* Sharp, focal kyphosis will be visible in the thoracic spine that is accentuated on forward bending (gibbus deformity) and is not reducible by thoracic hyperextension or by cervical extension during forward flexion. Forward flexion does not accentuate the kyphosis in postural kyphosis (no gibbus deformity), and the kyphosis is reduced with thoracic hyperextension or by extending the cervical spine during forward flexion.

- *Diagnostic Imaging.* Imaging should include upright PA, lateral and hyperextension views of the thoracic spine, as well as full cassette (36-inch) standing PA and lateral views of the entire spine to evaluate global balance. The criteria for diagnosing thoracic Scheuermann kyphosis include (1) thoracic kyphosis greater than 45 degrees, (2) at least 5 degrees of anterior wedging occurring in 3 or more adjacent vertebrae at the apex of the kyphosis, and (3) vertebral abnormalities including Schmorl's nodes, endplate irregularities, disc space narrowing, and AP vertebral elongation. These radiographic findings are not present in postural kyphosis. Scheuermann kyphosis is not reducible with hyperextension films whereas postural kyphosis should reduce during hyperextension radiographs.

References

1. Ginsburg GM, Bassett GS. Back pain in children and adolescents: evaluation and differential diagnosis. *J Am Acad Orthop Surg.* 1997;5:67-78.
2. Butler JS, Shelly MJ, Timlin M, Powderly WG, O'Byrne JM. Nontuberculous pyogenic spinal infection in adults: a 12-year experience from a tertiary referral center. *Spine.* 2006;31:2695-2700.
3. Wenger DR, Bobechko WP, Gilday DL. The spectrum of intervertebral disc-space infection in children. *J Bone Joint Surg Am.* 1978;60:100-108.
4. Lowe TG. Scheuermann's disease. *Orthop Clin North Am.* 1999;30:475-487, ix.

35

QUESTION

A 9-Year-Old Boy Came to the Emergency Room After Falling From a Tree. He Has a Lot of Neck Pain and Some Motor Weakness in his Upper and Lower Extremities. Is it Possible to Have Spinal Cord Injury Without Any Radiographic Abnormalities? How Should This Patient Be Managed?

Shay Bess, MD

SCIWORA (spinal cord injury without radiographic abnormality) is defined as a spinal cord injury (SCI) syndrome that does not demonstrate injury to the bony or ligamentous spinal column and does not demonstrate instability on plain film radiographs, computed tomography (CT), myelogram, or flexion/extension radiographs. This condition excludes injuries due to penetrating trauma, electrical shock, obstetric complications, and injuries associated with congenital spinal anomalies.[1] SCIWORA most commonly occurs in children aged 9 years and younger. This is likely because of the inherent flexibility and relative instability of the spinal column in this younger age group. This is especially true for the upper cervical spine (C2 to the occiput) in children. Similar to extremity injuries in this age group, the spine bends far beyond the normal physiologic range under traumatic conditions, but less commonly fractures. The neurological elements (spinal cord and nerve roots) must then incur the stress imparted to it by the hyperflexed or hyperextended spinal column. This concept is emphasized by neonatal cadaveric studies demonstrating that the spinal column is able to stretch up to 2 inches without damage; however, the spinal cord ruptures when stretched beyond 1/4 inch of forced lengthening.[2] This also explains why obstetric birth injuries associated with quadriplegia but no radiographic evidence of damage have demonstrated spinal cord rupture within an intact spinal column on autopsy examination. Beyond 12 years of age, the spinal column has similar biomechanics to that of an adult; consequently the bony elements will fracture and the ligamentous structures will rupture during traumatic conditions of forced hyperphysiologic range of motion. As such, SCI in patients aged 9 and younger will likely be without radiographic abnormality (SCIWORA), whereas SCI in patients older than 9 years will more likely be associated with a fracture, dislocation, and/or ligamentous disruption.

The most common level of SCIWORA injury occurs at the lower cervical spine (C5 distal). The majority of associated deficits are mild; however, approximately 22% of patients with SCIWORA are motor complete. Motor complete injuries are commonly associated with cord transection. The majority of the SCIWORA injuries with severe neurological deficit occur at the level of the upper cervical spine and more commonly occur in patients younger than 8 years of age. Consequently, SCIWORA must be considered in younger children that present with severe neurological deficits.

The term SCIWORA was coined before the advent of magnetic resonant imaging (MRI). Subsequent MRI imaging of patients diagnosed with SCIWORA has demonstrated multiple regions of abnormal signal intensity in the spinal column (anterior and posterior longitudinal ligament, annulus fibrosis, and facet capsules) as well as within the substance of the spinal cord. These findings on MRI combined with reported cases of delayed neurological deterioration and recurrent SCIWORA after an initial SCIWORA event have given rise to the concept of occult instability as the etiology of SCIWORA and have generated interest in the value of protecting an already injured spinal cord.

Neurological recovery is variable after a SCIWORA event. Complete recovery occurs in approximately 33%, partial recovery in 15%, and no recovery occurs in 49% of patients. Poor recovery prognosis is associated with severe neurological deficit and MRI findings consistent with cord transection or major cord hemorrhage (>50%). Mild to moderate neurological deficits, MRI findings indicative of minor cord hemorrhage (<50%), or cord edema only are associated with moderate to good recovery. The absence of abnormal cord signal change has suggested that the patient will have complete recovery.[3]

Figure 35-1 provides a diagnosis and treatment algorithm for pediatric patients with a suspected cervical spine injury.

References

1. Pang D. Spinal cord injury without radiographic abnormality in children, 2 decades later. *Neurosurgery.* 2004;55:1325-1342; discussion 1322-1343.
2. Leventhal HR. Birth injuries of the spinal cord. *J Pediatr.* 1960;56:447-453.
3. Launay F, Leet AI, Sponseller PD. Pediatric spinal cord injury without radiographic abnormality: a meta-analysis. *Clin Orthop Relat Res.* 2005;166-170.

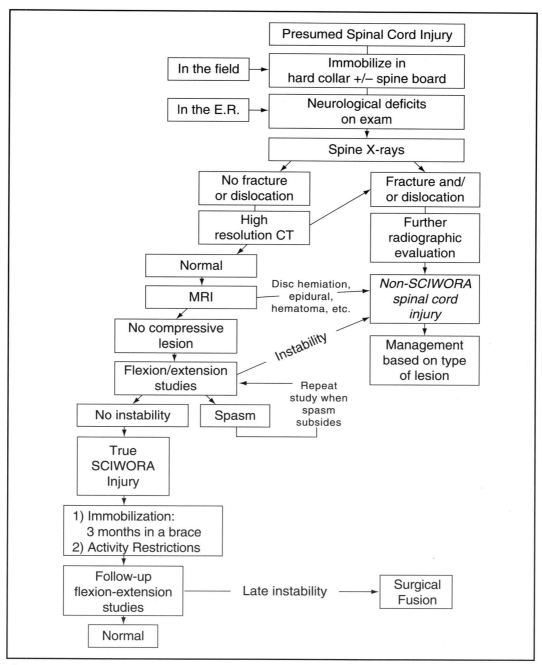

Figure 35-1. Management algorithm for pediatric cervical spine injuries. (Adapted from Pang D. Spinal cord injury without radiographic abnormality in children, 2 decades later. *Neurosurgery.* 2004;55:1325-1342.)

SECTION X

BONE GRAFTS

SOME OF MY PATIENTS COMPLAIN THAT THE ILIAC CREST BONE GRAFT SITE IS TENDER YEARS AFTER SURGERY. WHAT TYPES OF BONE GRAFT ALTERNATIVES ARE AVAILABLE FOR THE CERVICAL AND THORACOLUMBAR SPINE?

Shay Bess, MD

Despite a number of recent advances in bone grafting and bone graft substitutes, autogenous iliac crest bone graft (ICBG) remains the gold-standard fusion substrate for procedures in the cervical and thoracolumbar spine. However, often bone graft substitutes may necessary, and some important considerations are (1) the region of the spine to be fused (cervical, thoracic, or lumbar), (2) the column (anterior, posterior, or both) that will receive the fusion, and (3) the quality of the host.

It has been well reported that single and multilevel anterior interbody fusion in the cervical spine can be successfully performed using structural allograft when combined with an anterior plate.[1,2] Surgeons may elect to combine multilevel anterior cervical discectomy and fusion (ACDF) or multilevel cervical corpectomy with posterior spinal fusion when using allograft to increase fusion rates and to reduce the incidence of plate kickout or failure. Bone morphogenetic protein (BMP) has received a considerable amount of attention as a potential autograft substitute; however, the use of BMP (rhBMP-2, Infuse, Medtronic) in the anterior cervical spine has been associated with a number of complications related to anterior swelling, including respiratory distress and prolonged swallowing difficulties.[3,4] This is likely related to dose, because initial reports using a low dose of BMP in the cervical spine combined with structural allograft demonstrated high fusion and low complication rates. At the present time, BMP is an off-label use in the cervical spine and in strongly discouraged by the manufacturer. There are fewer reports describing use of polyetheretherketone (PEEK) or titanium mesh cages in the anterior cervical

Figure 36-1. Bone graft substitutes. Femoral ring allograft (FRA) used for anterior lumbar interbody fusion (ALIF) in conjunction with an instrumented posterior spinal fusion to generate an anteroposterior spinal fusion (APSF) or 360-degree fusion. The benefit of FRA is that it provides structural interbody support (unlike morselized autograft) and will act as a scaffold for a biological product (autograft, demineralized bone matrix, bone morphogenetic protein, etc) to promote interbody fusion.

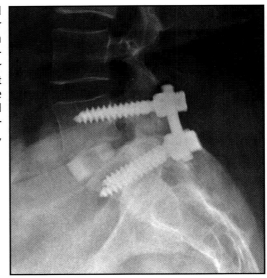

interspace in combination with bone marrow aspirate and morselized allograft or ceramics (beta-tricalcium phosphate).

Traditionally, a posterior cervical fusion is performed using posterior ICBG; however, morselized allograft can be packed into the decorticated facets and over the posterior elements. Alternatively, a structural allograft can be wired to the posterior elements or between the spinous processes. I prefer to use structural allograft in the anterior column with an anterior plate and use posterior ICBG, local bone graft, or structural iliac crest autograft for posterior spinal fusion (especially for C1-2 posterior fusion).

The question of the host and anterior versus posterior column grafting is particularly important in the thoracolumbar spine. Bone graft substitutes are more successful in the anterior column because they are loaded in compression, creating a favorable environment for fusion. However, the posterior column is loaded in tension, creating a challenging environment for onlay bone graft. Traditionally, allograft has underperformed in the thoracolumbar spine. That being said, Betz et al[5] showed the importance of the host when selecting a graft material. The authors reported no difference in fusion rates among 76 adolescent patients treated with instrumented posterior spinal fusion (PSF) for adolescent idiopathic scoliosis (AIS) who were randomized to either allograft or no grafting material.[5] Femoral ring allograft or structural cages (PEEK and titanium) are readily accepted implants for the anterior column in the thoracolumbar spine (Figure 36-1). These implants have traditionally been filled with morselized autograft. Initial data using BMP with structural allograft and titanium cages have demonstrated excellent results with faster healing rates, greater fusion rates, and reduced harvest site morbidity than cages filled with autograft.[6]

As mentioned, posterior and posterolateral fusion in the adult thoracolumbar spine has remained a challenge even when using ICBG. One-level instrumented lumbar fusion using local bone has demonstrated equal clinical and radiographic results to fusions supplemented with ICBG. However, solid arthrodesis in multilevel fusions is more difficult, especially in older patients that have less autograft available for harvest. The success of BMP in the anterior column has motivated further research into using BMP in the posterior column. Two forms of BMP are available for use in the posterior spine. BMP-7 (OP-1, Stryker) is approved by the Food and Drug Administration (FDA) for use in single- or multilevel lumbar fusion in hosts who present a challenge to achieving solid arthrodesis (revision for demonstrated nonunion, multiple medical comorbidities, smoker, for example).[7] BMP-2 is currently not FDA approved for use in the posterior spine. Initial data for both of these substances as autograft replacements are encouraging. The higher BMP doses (and thus higher cost) required in the posterior spine make BMP use less attractive. Bone marrow aspirate applied to either a collagen sponge or morselized bone graft has demonstrated promising results in the posterior column. I prefer to use BMP with a structural cage (PEEK or allograft) in the anterior column and use local bone with ICBG posterolaterally for thoracolumbar fusions. Allograft is usually an excellent autograft graft substitute for posterior thoracolumbar fusions in AIS. For multilevel thoracolumbar fusions in the adult patient, I prefer to supplement the posterior fusion with BMP and allograft.

References

1. Samartzis D, Shen FH, Matthews DK, Yoon ST, Goldberg EJ, An HS. Comparison of allograft to autograft in multilevel anterior cervical discectomy and fusion with rigid plate fixation. *Spine.* 2003;3:451-459.
2. Samartzis D, Shen FH, Goldberg EJ, An HS. Is autograft the gold standard in achieving radiographic fusion in one-level anterior cervical discectomy and fusion with rigid anterior plate fixation? *Spine.* 2005;30:1756-1761.
3. Smucker JD, Rhee JM, Singh K, Yoon ST, Heller JG. Increased swelling complications associated with off-label usage of rhBMP-2 in the anterior cervical spine. *Spine.* 2006;31:2813-2819.
4. Shields LB, Raque GH, Glassman SD, et al. Adverse effects associated with high-dose recombinant human bone morphogenetic protein-2 use in anterior cervical spine fusion. *Spine.* 2006;31:542-547.
5. Betz RR, Petrizzo AM, Kerner PJ, Falatyn SP, Clements DH, Huss GK. Allograft versus no graft with a posterior multisegmented hook system for the treatment of idiopathic scoliosis. *Spine.* 2006;31:121-127.
6. Burkus JK, Gornet MF, Dickman CA, Zdeblick TA. Anterior lumbar interbody fusion using rhBMP-2 with tapered interbody cages. *J Spinal Disord Tech.* 2002;15:337-349.
7. Vaccaro AR, Patel T, Fischgrund J, et al. A pilot study evaluating the safety and efficacy of OP-1 Putty (rhBMP-7) as a replacement for iliac crest autograft in posterolateral lumbar arthrodesis for degenerative spondylolisthesis. *Spine.* 2004;29:1885-1892.

SECTION XI

INTRAOPERATIVE

37

DO I NEED TO PERFORM NEUROMONITORING FOR EVERY SPINE SURGERY? THE COST IS RELATIVELY HIGH AND I WANT TO BE SELECTIVE ABOUT ITS USE.

Shay Bess, MD

The question of when to perform neuromonitoring depends upon the surgical risks that may be encountered during the procedure.[1] The most commonly used modalities include spontaneous and triggered electromyography (EMG), somatosensory-evoked potentials (SSEPs), and motor-evoked potentials (MEPs). Triggered and spontaneous EMGs are used to test nerve root function and irritation. Spinal cord function is monitored using SSEPs (evaluating the integrity of the ascending sensory pathways) and MEPs (evaluating the integrity of the descending motor pathways). EMGs can be run throughout the procedure and give immediate feedback. MEPs will also give nearly immediate feedback, whereas SSEPs require signal averaging and require several minutes for response. The theoretical benefit of neurological monitoring is that the surgeon may be warned of an eminent neurological complication and may be able to take corrective action before the event becomes irreversible. However, a number of studies have demonstrated false negative readings that give the surgeon a false sense of security. Other studies have demonstrated false positive readings that may motivate the surgeon to take unnecessary corrective action or may create undue stress during the procedure. Consequently, the complication rates of each procedure must be evaluated in light of these false positive and false negative rates.

Nerve root complications are more common than spinal cord complications (10% vs 0.3%, respectively) during spine surgery. Accordingly, the use of EMGs to detect potential nerve root injuries during the procedure is a valuable modality. EMG monitoring is carried out in two fashions, spontaneous and triggered. Spontaneous EMGs are a real-time recording of EMG activity that detects nerve root action potentials. This may reflect nerve root irritation due to mechanical insult or positioning. Therefore, the surgeon may be notified of an occurring insult, rather than notification of nerve root dysfunction once an injury has occurred. However, spontaneous EMG activity occurs during a high percentage of procedures and has been shown to have a poor correlation with neurological outcome. Triggered EMGs are a compound motor action potential in response to a stimulated nerve root. The most common use for triggered EMGs includes pedicle screw stimulation or pedicle screw tract probing and stimulation to detect a potential pedicle screw tract breech. EMGs will be suppressed by neuromuscular blockade. Accurate EMG readings require neuromuscular blockade be at least partially reversed (2 or more twitches on anesthesia motor stimulation).

Spinal cord monitoring during spinal deformity surgery (scoliosis, kyphosis) is currently an accepted standard and should be utilized during all deformity surgery, especially when performed on the thoracic spine. Studies released by the Scoliosis Research Society (SRS) demonstrated a 60% reduction in paralysis and paraparesis when using SSEP monitoring for deformity surgery.[2-4] MEPs are a relatively new monitoring technique and therefore have less support in the literature; however, studies have reported that MEPs have a higher sensitivity and specificity to detect motor deficits than SSEPs. Another benefit of MEPs as compared to SSEPs is that MEP monitoring has a markedly shorter latent period from the onset of the deficit to the appearance of an abnormality during monitoring.[5] Spinal cord monitoring is progressively becoming more routine during spine tumor resection (intra- and extramedullary) and during thoracolumbar trauma surgery in patients who are neurologically intact and/or have incomplete neurological deficits. It should be noted that SSEPs and MEPs are affected by anesthetic agents (especially inhalational agents) and by hypotension; therefore the surgeon must keep in mind that a loss of SSEPs or MEPs may be a reflection of the anesthesia that is being used or of a hypotensive event rather than a cord injury. These possibilities must be kept in the forefront of the differential diagnosis and ruled out initially when an abnormality in SSEP or MEP monitoring is reported.

Because of the possibility of spinal cord injury during thoracic deformity, thoracic trauma, and tumor surgery, and because of the unquestionable value of neurological monitoring, I use a combination of EMGs, SSEPs, and MEPs during these cases. I also use a combination of spontaneous EMGs, SSEPs, and MEPs during cervical decompression for patients with myelopathy, for patients who have traumatic or pathologic cord compression, and during correction of cervical deformity. I also use these modalities when performing a cervical corpectomy.[5,6]

When performing instrumented lumbar fusion surgery below the level of the conus, I use spontaneous EMGs throughout the case and use triggered EMGs to test the pedicle screws.

Because of the relatively high incidence of false positive and false negative rates when using EMGs during surgery for cervical and lumbar radiculopathy I do not use neurological monitoring during anterior cervical discectomy and fusion for cervical radiculopathy, lumbar discectomy, or lumbar decompression for lumbar spinal stenosis. For many authors, the financial and emotional cost outweighs the benefits of EMG monitoring in these cases.[7]

References

1. Slimp J. Intraoperative neurophysiological monitoring of the spinal cord and nerve roots. *SpineLine.* 2006;7:6-15.
2. Nuwer MR, Dawson EG, Carlson LG, Kanim LE, Sherman JE. Somatosensory evoked potential spinal cord monitoring reduces neurologic deficits after scoliosis surgery: results of a large multicenter survey. *Electroencephalogr Clin Neurophysiol.* 1995;96:6-11.
3. Dawson EG, Sherman JE, Kanim LE, Nuwer MR. Spinal cord monitoring: results of the Scoliosis Research Society and the European Spinal Deformity Society survey. *Spine.* 1991;16:S361-364.
4. Padberg AM, Wilson-Holden TJ, Lenke LG, Bridwell KH. Somatosensory- and motor-evoked potential monitoring without a wake-up test during idiopathic scoliosis surgery: an accepted standard of care. *Spine.* 1998;23:1392-1400.
5. Hilibrand AS, Schwartz DM, Sethuraman V, Vaccaro AR, Albert TJ. Comparison of transcranial electric motor and somatosensory evoked potential monitoring during cervical spine surgery. *J Bone Joint Surg Am.* 2004;86-A:1248-1253.
6. Khan MH, Smith PN, Balzer JR, et al. Intraoperative somatosensory evoked potential monitoring during cervical spine corpectomy surgery: experience with 508 cases. *Spine.* 2006;31:E105-113.
7. Smith PN, Balzer JR, Khan MH, et al. Intraoperative somatosensory evoked potential monitoring during anterior cervical discectomy and fusion in nonmyelopathic patients—a review of 1,039 cases. *Spine.* 2007;7:83-87.

SECTION XII

POSTOPERATIVE PATIENTS

QUESTION 38

WHEN SHOULD I BRACE MY THORACOLUMBAR FUSIONS?

Shay Bess, MD

Very little data exist to support or refute the value of bracing after thoracolumbar (TL) fusion.[1,2] No study to date has demonstrated increased fusion rates, reduced instrumentation failure, reduced screw-bone interface failure, or improved clinical outcomes when patients are braced following TL fusion compared to patients that are not braced. Consequently, the only guidelines for postoperative bracing are empiric data based upon surgeon training and preference. In general, the rationale for bracing a patient following TL fusion can be roughly divided into four categories: (1) to provide additional stability to promote fusion, (2) to protect spinal instrumentation, (3) to provide external support for acute postoperative pain control, and (4) to ensure patient and/or care provider compliance with postoperative activity restrictions.

When using a brace as insurance to protect a long instrumented construct, to protect a construct in osteoporotic bone, or when used postoperatively for traumatic conditions that have reduced anterior column support or ligamentous damage, the best bracing option is likely a rigid orthosis, either a lumbosacral orthosis (LSO, used for fusions that extend up to L2) or a thoracolumbosacral orthosis (TLSO, used fusions that extend cephalad to L2 to approximately T7) (Figure 38-1). Orthotists often divide rigid braces into either custom fitted (standard "off the shelf" brace that is modified to fit the patient) or custom molded braces (the brace is created specifically for the patient using a plaster of Paris mold). The obvious benefit of the rigid braces is more external support than flexible braces.[3] Some data suggest that external orthoses minimally reduce postoperative spinal segmental motion.[4] Furthermore, to effectively reduce motion at the lumbosacral junction, a spica cast or thigh addition must be added to the brace.[3,4] Rigid braces also have a propensity for causing skin breakdown and creating decubitus ulcers, especially if the patient is asked to sleep in the brace. Consequently, patients should be vigilant about skin care when using rigid braces, especially a molded LSO or TLSO. The patient should remain in close contact with the fitting orthotist so that alterations to the brace can be made to remove or pad areas that create skin irritation. Rigid braces are also poorly tolerated during warm weather and may reduce patient compliance.

Patients may have poor paraspinal muscle control following TL surgery because of tissue dissection and may benefit from a custom fitted brace or a less rigid lumbosacral corset.

Figure 38-1. Custom molded thoracolumbosacral orthosis (TLSO). This brace is created specifically for the patient using a plaster mold. A TLSO has multiple uses including postoperative bracing following spinal fusion, nonoperative treatment for spinal fractures, and brace treatment for childhood scoliosis.

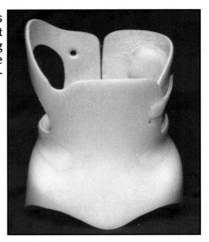

These braces may offer some pain relief in the acute postoperative period by providing temporary external support.

When using a brace to ensure patient compliance with postoperative activity modifications, the surgeon must consider that although the brace may act as a reminder for the patient or caregivers to avoid vigorous movement or activity, if a patient will not be compliant with postoperative activity modification, the patient most likely will also not be compliant with brace wear. Consequently, the patient's family or caregivers must also be included in the discussion as to why the brace is being used and the rationale behind the postoperative activity modifications.

Because of the lack of good data supporting or refuting the benefits of bracing following TL fusion, I prefer not to use a postoperative brace. If the patient is reporting postoperative postural pain during ambulation or physical therapy, I will use a custom fitted LSO/TLSO or lumbosacral corset for temporary pain control. I encourage the patient to wear the brace for only approximately 3 to 6 weeks, so that the brace does not interfere with postoperative physical therapy and cause abdominal and paraspinal muscle atrophy. If the patient is beginning to develop postoperative proximal junctional kyphosis, if the surgery was performed for kyphogenic pathology, or if the TL fusion was performed for a traumatic condition and the anterior column support is compromised, I will attempt to use a custom molded brace to control the kyphosis. It should be noted that there is absolutely no data to support this. If I am concerned that the patient will not be compliant with postoperative activity modification (especially for patients undergoing TL fusion for traumatic conditions or infection), I will use a custom fitted or custom molded brace, with the understanding that the brace may spend most of the time on the floor rather than on the patient.

References

1. Resnick DK, Choudhri TF, Dailey AT, et al. Guidelines for the performance of fusion procedures for degenerative disease of the lumbar spine, part 14: brace therapy as an adjunct to or substitute for lumbar fusion. *J Neurosurg Spine.* 2005;2:716-724.
2. Connolly PJ, Grob D. Bracing of patients after fusion for degenerative problems of the lumbar spine—yes or no? *Spine.* 1998;23:1426-1428.
3. Fidler MW, Plasmans CM. The effect of four types of support on the segmental mobility of the lumbosacral spine. *J Bone Joint Surg Am.* 1983;65:943-947.
4. Axelsson P, Johnsson R, Stromqvist B. Effect of lumbar orthosis on intervertebral mobility: a roentgen stereophotogrammetric analysis. *Spine.* 1992;17:678-681.

SECTION XIII

SPORTS MEDICINE

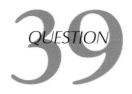

I WAS AT A HIGH SCHOOL FOOTBALL GAME WHEN I SAW A FOOTBALL PLAYER ATTEMPT TO SPEAR-TACKLE ANOTHER PLAYER; HIS ARMS AND LEGS TEMPORARILY BECAME NUMB. WHAT HAPPENED TO THAT PLAYER AND HOW SHOULD HE BE FOLLOWED?

Shay Bess, MD

Neurapraxia of the cervical spinal cord with transient quadriparesis or quadriplegia occurs in approximately 7 per 10,000 mature football players.[1] The incidence of cervical neurapraxia (CN) in younger football players and in athletes participating in other sports is unknown. The mechanism of injury includes forced hyperflexion or hyperextension of the cervical spine, most often occurring when the athlete initiates contact with the head (ie, spear-tackling or head butting). Symptoms include temporary burning in the upper and lower extremities, loss of sensation, and/or loss of motor function. Motor recovery is most commonly seen within 15 minutes; however, sensory changes may persist for several days.[2] The mechanism of injury is theorized to be a result of forced cervical hyperflexion or hyperextension that reduces the spinal canal diameter and compresses the cervical spinal cord by a "pincer" mechanism, resulting in transient spinal cord dysfunction. Athletes with congenital cervical stenosis (CCS) as measured by the Pavlov/Torg ratio (lateral spinal canal to lateral vertebral body ratio; Figure 39-1) are at an increased risk for CN. The normal Pavlov/Torg ratio is 1. Athletes with a Pavlov/Torg ratio less than or equal to 0.8 are defined as having CCS and have an increased incidence of CN.[3] The Pavlov/Torg ratio is helpful when predicting recurrent episodes of CN; however, it is a

Figure 39-1. Pavlov/Torg ratio or spinal canal–vertebral body ratio. Measured by the distance from the midpoint of the posterior aspect of the vertebral body to the nearest point on the corresponding spinolaminar line (a) divided by the anteroposterior width of the vertebral body (b). The normal ratio is 1. Ratio for congenital cervical stenosis is less than or equal to 0.8.

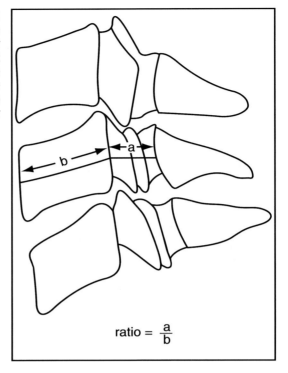

$$\text{ratio} = \frac{a}{b}$$

poor screening tool when initially evaluating athletes because of the demonstrated poor predictive value for CN and other athletic injuries.[4] Consequently, much debate exists as to the appropriate application of the Pavlov/Torg ratio.[5]

All patients with CN should be managed similar to patients with an unstable spine injury. Regardless of the rapidity of neurologic recovery, initial care involves spine immobilization and emergency transport to a hospital facility with magnetic resonant imaging (MRI) capacity. Evaluation in the hospital should include a thorough neurological evaluation; plain film radiographs of the cervical, thoracic, and lumbar spine; and MRI of the cervical spine. As indicated previously, if there is no structural damage to the bony or ligamentous cervical spine, symptoms usually resolve in majority of patients within 2 days. The guidelines for return to play remain controversial. There are few reports indicating permanent neurological deficits after a recurrent episode of CN. However, Torg et al indicated that athletes with CCS who have suffered one previous episode of CN represent a relative contraindication to return play. Athletes who have had 2 or more episodes of CN or have neurological symptoms or deficits that last more than 36 hours should not return to competition (Table 39-1).[2]

The incidence of CN in younger athletes is not known, and no correlation has been established for CCS and CN in pediatric athletes. Consequently, no guidelines exist for return to play for immature athletes who suffer a CN event. However, because of the relative ligamentous laxity and increased cervical range of motion in the pediatric cervical spine, many guidelines mandate that a single episode of CN in an immature athlete represents an absolute contraindication for return to play.[5]

Table 39-1

Guidelines for Return to Play for an Athlete Who Sustained Previous Cervical Neurapraxia

No contraindication to participation	Spinal canal-vertebral body ratio 0.8 in an asymptomatic individual who has never had an event of cervical neurapraxia
Relative contraindication	1. Spinal canal-vertebral body ratio 0.8 with 1 episode of cervical neurapraxia 2. Documented episode of cervical neurapraxia associated with intervertebral disc disease and/or degenerative changes 3. Documented episode of cervical neurapraxia associated with MRI evidence of cord deformation
Absolute contraindication	1. Documented episode of cervical cord neurapraxia associated with MRI evidence of cord defect or cord edema 2. Documented episode of cervical cord neurapraxia associated with ligamentous instability, neurologic symptoms lasting more than 36 hours, and/or multiple episodes

References

1. Torg JS, Pavlov H, Genuario SE, et al. Neurapraxia of the cervical spinal cord with transient quadriplegia. *J Bone Joint Surg Am.* 1986;68:1354-1370.
2. Torg JS, Guille JT, Jaffe S. Injuries to the cervical spine in American football players. *J Bone Joint Surg Am.* 2002;84-A:112-122.
3. Pavlov H, Torg JS, Robie B, Jahre C. Cervical spinal stenosis: determination with vertebral body ratio method. *Radiology.* 1987;164:771-775.
4. Torg JS, Naranja RJ Jr, Pavlov H, Galinat BJ, Warren R, Stine RA. The relationship of developmental narrowing of the cervical spinal canal to reversible and irreversible injury of the cervical spinal cord in football players. *J Bone Joint Surg Am.* 1996;78:1308-1314.
5. Herman MJ. Cervical spine injuries in the pediatric and adolescent athlete. *Instr Course Lect.* 2006;55:641-646.

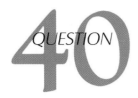

WHAT IS A BURNER/STINGER AND HOW SHOULD IT BE MANAGED?

Shay Bess, MD

A burner or stinger injury is a transitory brachial plexus injury (transient brachial plexopathy) caused by forced stretching of the head and neck toward or away from the affected limb, resulting in excessive traction or compression on the brachial plexus. Brachial plexopathy injuries most often occur in contact sports when the athlete leads with his or her head to initiate contact or sustains a blow that results in forced lateral extension away from or forced compression toward the affected limb (Figure 40-1).[1] Symptoms include burning paresthetic pain and numbness that radiates into the affected limb with associated transitory weakness. The diagnosis is easily made because the athlete will often appear after the contact event holding and shaking the affected arm. The athlete should immediately be removed from the playing field for evaluation. Classically, the athlete will report that he or she had a "dead arm" after the inciting event.

Physical examination should include a mental status evaluation to rule out an associated head injury. The cervical spine is then palpated for midline and paracervical tenderness and/or bony step-offs. A thorough motor and sensory examination should be preformed to elucidate the presence of a neurological deficit and should serve as a baseline for persistent or resolved symptoms. A preganglionic injury (representing nerve root avulsion proximal to the dorsal root ganglion) should be ruled out by inspecting for loss of sensation proximal to the clavicle, Horner syndrome (ptosis, miosis, and anhydrosis of the ipsilateral eye), and scapular winging. This is followed by a Spurling test, which involves rotating and laterally tilting the head toward the symptomatic extremity. A positive Spurling test will recreate the pain and is indicative of nerve root irritation (Figure 40-2).

Sensory and motor function commonly returns shortly after the event, and most symptoms resolve within 10 minutes.[2] The motor and sensory examination should be repeated when symptoms resolve. If the symptoms resolve quickly and there is no associated cervical spine tenderness, no acute treatment is necessary. The condition must be differentiated from cervical neurapraxia, which is a cervical cord contusion syndrome.

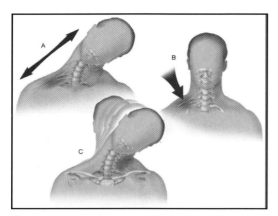

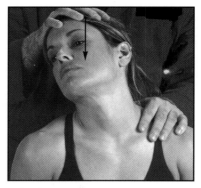

Figure 40-1. Injury mechanism for transient brachial plexopathy. Forced motion of the head and neck away from or toward the affected limb can generate a traction or compressive injury to the brachial plexus and associated plexopathy.

Figure 40-2. Spurling maneuver. Head rotation and lateral tilt toward the symptomatic extremity recreate the radicular extremity pain by reducing the size of the neural foramen and compressing the nerve root within foramen. A positive Spurling test (recreation of the extremity pain) is indicative of nerve root irritation and associated radiculopathy.

Return to play following a transient brachial plexopathy has become somewhat controversial. Most guidelines allow return to play when the athlete is asymptomatic and the physical examination is normal.[3] Athletes who are persistently symptomatic or have a neurological examination that remains abnormal should be withheld from competition. The severity of the injury is graded according to the severity and duration of symptoms.

Recurrent burners are problematic for many athletes and may contraindicate return to competition. Athletes with congenital cervical stenosis as determined by a Pavlov/Torg ratio less than or equal to 0.8 (width of the lateral spinal canal to lateral vertebral body ratio) are at risk for recurrent burners. However, congenital cervical stenosis should not be used as a screening tool because of the low positive predictive value for transitory brachial plexopathy and cervical cord neurapraxia. Athletes who have recurrent burners often have a positive Spurling test that recreates the arm symptoms associated with the burners. MRI examinations of athletes who have recurrent burners demonstrate a high incidence of foraminal stenosis and cervical degenerative disease. Athletes who experience 1 or 2 burner episodes may return to play when symptoms have completely resolved.[4] These athletes should use protective equipment. Athletes who suffer 3 burner episodes should be excluded from competition because of the high risk of recurrent episodes and continued risk for permanent injury.

References

1. Herman MJ. Cervical spine injuries in the pediatric and adolescent athlete. *Instr Course Lect.* 2006;55:641-646.
2. Kasow DB, Curl WW. "Stingers" in adolescent athletes. *Instr Course Lect.* 2006;55:711-716.
3. Vaccaro AR, Watkins B, Albert TJ, Pfaff WL, Klein GR, Silber JS. Cervical spine injuries in athletes: current return-to-play criteria. *Orthopedics.* 2001;24:699-703.
4. Weinberg J, Rokito S, Silber JS. Etiology, treatment, and prevention of athletic "stingers." *Clin Sports Med.* 2003;22:493-500, viii.

SECTION XIV

DEFORMITY

I HAVE A 34-YEAR-OLD MALE WITH GRADE III SPONDYLOLISTHESIS. SHOULD I FUSE THE PATIENT IN SITU OR SHOULD I ATTEMPT A REDUCTION?

Yu-Po Lee, MD

The term spondylolisthesis is derived from the Greek words spondylos (vertebra) and olithesis (slip). These terms most commonly describe the forward slippage of one vertebra on another. The classification schemes by Wiltse[1] and Meyerding are the most widely accepted classifications of spondylolisthesis (Tables 41-1 and 41-2).

For adults, the surgical indications are persistent back pain and neurologic or radicular symptoms unresponsive to nonoperative treatment. Neurogenic claudication and radicular symptoms are more responsive than back pain to surgery.

Treating a patient with a high-grade spondylolisthesis can be very challenging, and opinions vary as to the best form of management. The patient described in this question most likely has an isthmic spondylolisthesis at L5-S1. Some authors have reported good results with an isolated posterior fusion in situ.[2,3] However, pseudoarthrosis rates have been reported to be as high as 44%, and progression is common, even with a radiographically solid fusion. In addition, fusion in situ fails to correct the clinical deformity and sagittal imbalance that generally accompany these severe deformities.

On the other hand, instrumentation and reduction of a grade III spondylolisthesis can be technically challenging, and there is a greater risk of nerve root injury with the reduction, typically involving the fifth lumbar root.[4] This neuropraxia can result in a foot drop, and patients often have only partial recovery. The addition of an anterior interbody fusion is also controversial. Although some series report good results with isolated posterior spinal fusion, others report higher fusion rates, less progression, and fewer implant failures with circumferential fusion. However, the benefits of adding an anterior interbody fusion must be weighed against the increased morbidity of the anterior procedure, which includes nerve and vessel injury and a 0 to 4% risk of retrograde ejaculation in males if the superior hypogastric plexus is injured.

Taking all of these factors into consideration, I would recommend an anterior reduction and interbody fusion at L5-S1 with a posterolateral fusion augmented with pedicle screws

Table 41-1

Wiltse Classification of Spondylolisthesis[1]

Type	Name	Description
I	Congenital	Dysplastic abnormalities in posterior elements or the upper sacrum.
II	Isthmic	Secondary to defect in the pars interarticularis. There are three types: A. Lytic, presumed to be a stress fracture of the pars B. Elongation of the pars w/o separation (possibly a healed fracture) C. Acute fracture of the pars interarticularis from high-energy trauma
III	Degenerative	Neural arch is intact. The slippage results from segmental instability.
IV	Traumatic	Fracture other than the pars interarticularis resulting in slippage.
V	Postsurgical	Iatrogenic slippage as a result of loss of the posterior elements secondary to surgery.

Table 41-2

Meyerding Classification of Spondylolisthesis Grade

Grade I	0 to 25% slippage		Grade IV	75 to 100%
Grade II	25 to 50%		Grade V	>100% (spondyloptosis)
Grade III	50 to 75%			

from L4-S1. The benefits of this plan include an indirect decompression at the neuroforamen, improved sagittal balance, and improved fusion rates. We hope the indirect anterior decompression, along with a posterior decompression if needed, will adequately treat the neurologic symptoms this patient is experiencing. Furthermore, a stable fusion will provide the patient with long-term relief. Studies have shown that a solid fusion was the main parameter that improves patient outcome. I am choosing to fuse to L4 in this situation because this helps to distribute the stress across the L4 and L5 levels. Iliosacral screws may be considered in this situation. I chose not to use them here as I was able to get a large femoral ring allograft strut anteriorly along with solid sacral fixation posteriorly. If my S1 screws were suboptimal, I would augment my construct with iliosacral screws (Figures 41-1A to D).

References

1. Wiltse, LL, Winter, RB. Terminology and measurement of spondylolisthesis. *J Bone Joint Surg (Am)*. 1983;65:768-772.
2. Remes V, Lamberg T, Tervahartiala P, et al. Long-term outcome after posterolateral, anterior, and circumferential fusion for high-grade isthmic spondylolisthesis in children and adolescents: magnetic resonance imaging findings after average of 17-year follow-up. *Spine*. 2006;31(21):2491-2499.
3. Helenius I, Lamberg T, Osterman K, et al. Posterolateral, anterior, or circumferential fusion in situ for high-grade spondylolisthesis in young patients: a long-term evaluation using the Scoliosis Research Society questionnaire. *Spine*. 2006;31(2):190-196.
4. DeWald CJ, Vartabedian JE, Rodts MF, et al. Evaluation and management of high-grade spondylolisthesis in adults. *Spine*. 2005;30(6 Suppl):S49-59.

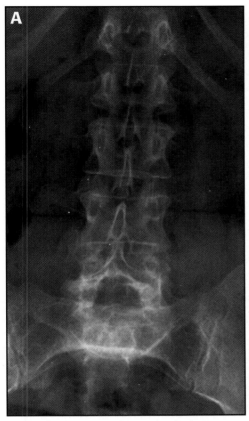

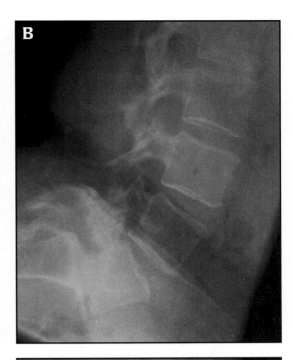

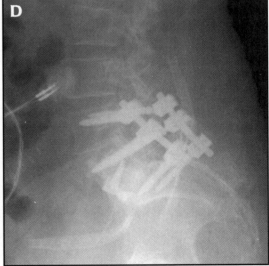

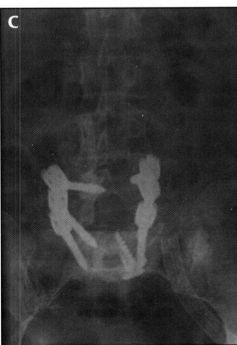

Figure 41-1. (A, B) AP and lateral preoperative radiographs demonstrating a Grade III spondylolisthesis. (C, D) Postoperative radiographs demonstrating femoral ring allograft at L5-S1 with pedicle screw instrumentation from L4-S1.

42

I HAVE A 16-YEAR-OLD FEMALE AND A 76-YEAR-OLD FEMALE WITH SCOLIOSIS. IS EVERY SCOLIOSIS THE SAME OR ARE THERE DIFFERENT TYPES?

Yu-Po Lee, MD

There are actually many different types of scoliosis. Scoliosis is by definition a curvature of the spine measuring greater than 10 degrees in the coronal plane. However, it must be kept in mind that scoliosis is truly a three-dimensional disease, and sagittal balance must also be taken into account when treating these patients.

In skeletally immature patients, there are many types of scoliosis. These include congenital, idiopathic, and neuromuscular scoliosis. In skeletally mature patients, prior idiopathic scoliosis and de novo degenerative scoliosis are the most common forms. Less common types include congenital deformities that present in adulthood, paralytic curves, posttraumatic deformities, iatrogenic deformities, and curves related to severe osteoporosis. In the following discussion, I primarily limit my discussion to congenital, idiopathic, and degenerative scoliosis.

Congenital scoliosis is a coronal imbalance of the spine caused by vertebral anomalies. These anomalies arise during weeks 4 to 6 of the embryonic period while the vertebrae are forming, but the curvature may take years to become clinically evident. Congenital scoliosis can be divided into defects of segmentation and defects of formation. However, some congenital abnormalities may not fit into either one of these categories. In defects of segmentation, the subtypes include a block vertebra, unilateral bar, and unilateral bar with a hemivertebra. The subtypes of defects of formation include hemivertebra and wedge vertebra. Patients with a unilateral segmented bar with a contralateral hemivertebra and those with a unilateral unsegmented bar are the most likely to progress (Figure 42-1A).

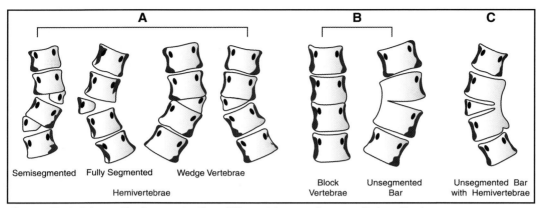

Figure 42-1. Schematic demonstrating different types of congenital scoliosis.

Congenital anomalies are frequently associated with other organ system disorders. It has been reported that approximately 50% of patients have an associated organ defect. The most common systems affected are the cardiac and renal systems. Hence, these patients should have a screening renal ultrasound and cardiac evaluation including an echocardiogram prior to surgery. Intraspinal abnormalities are also common. Up to 38% of patients with congenital vertebral anomalies have intraspinal anomalies that include tethered cord, diastematomyelia, diplomyelia, and syringomyelia. Vertebral anomalies occur with a constellation of other defects 38% to 55% of the time to form VATER syndrome. The presence of vertebral anomalies, anorectal anomalies, tracheoesophageal fistula, and renal and vascular anomalies form the VATER syndrome. The presence of vertebral anomalies, anorectal anomalies, tracheoesophageal fistula, and renal and vascular anomalies together with cardiac and limb defects are known as the VACTERL syndrome. The role of bracing is limited in congenital scoliosis because many of these deformities are rigid, and surgery depends on the type and location of the anomaly.

Idiopathic scoliosis is divided into infantile, juvenile, and adolescent depending on the age of onset. Infantile idiopathic scoliosis is diagnosed in patients who present before the age of 3, juvenile idiopathic scoliosis is diagnosed in patients who present between 4 and 9 years of age, and adolescent idiopathic scoliosis is diagnosed in patients who present after age 10. Infantile idiopathic scoliosis constitutes less than 1% of all idiopathic scoliosis and has been shown to resolve in more than 90% of patients spontaneously. It is more common in males and typically is left sided (75% to 90%). Poor prognosis is noted in boys with right-sided thoracic curves. The rib-vertebra angle has been the most reliable prognostic indicator of curve progression.

Adolescent idiopathic scoliosis is the most common form of scoliosis seen in children and is seen in 1% to 3% of the population.[1] The natural history depends on several factors including the degree of skeletal maturity, curve magnitude, curve location, and curve pattern. In the past, the King-Moe classification was used, but the Lenke classification system has become increasingly more popular.[1] Treatment is based on observation, orthoses, and surgery depending upon the type and magnitude of the curve. Surgery is performed to correct the deformity and then to fuse the spine once correction has been achieved. This can be done anteriorly, posteriorly, or combined depending upon the type and magnitude of the curve as well as surgeon preference. I prefer a posterior approach and the use of pedicle screws. Very good results have been seen with pedicle screws as they are biomechanically superior to hooks.[2,3] Also, with pedicle screws, it is easier to maintain sagittal alignment and avoid creating a flatback deformity. For curves greater than 75 degrees, I would consider a combined approach.

Adult scoliosis is generally related to prior idiopathic scoliosis and de novo degenerative scoliosis. The clinical presentation is somewhat different than for adolescents. Older patients often have increasing back pain or progressive trunk imbalance. Some patients may also report neurogenic claudication from stenosis. The primary indications for surgery are a progressive deformity, the development of poor spinal balance causing functional difficulties, a large deformity threatening cardiopulmonary compromise, or the presence of neurologic deficits.

References

1. Lenke LG, Betz RR, Harms J, et al. Adolescent idiopathic scoliosis: a new classification to determine extent of spinal arthrodesis. *J Bone Joint Surg Am.* 2001;83-A(8):1169-1181.
2. Kim YJ, Bridwell KH, Lenke LG, et al. Pseudarthrosis in long adult spinal deformity instrumentation and fusion to the sacrum: prevalence and risk factor analysis of 144 cases. *Spine.* 2006;31(20):2329-2336.
3. Kim YJ, Lenke LG, Kim J, et al. Comparative analysis of pedicle screw versus hybrid instrumentation in posterior spinal fusion of adolescent idiopathic scoliosis. *Spine.* 2006;31(3):291-298.

I Have a 13-Year-Old Girl With a Progressive Thoracolumbar Curve That Has Been Refractory to Bracing. When Is Surgery Indicated in Adolescent Idiopathic Scoliosis?

Yu-Po Lee, MD

Surgical decision making in adolescent idiopathic scoliosis is based on the probability that a curve will progress and the anticipated effect of the deformity on the patient into adulthood. Two important variables that predict curve progression include the magnitude and type of curve. Multiple studies have shown that the larger the curve at the first visit, the more rapid the progression. The type of curve also may affect progression, with thoracic curves more likely to progress than lumbar curves, although lumbar curves are more likely to progress and cause problems in adulthood. In general, double-curve patterns progress more rapidly than single-curve patterns.[1]

Another important variable is where the child is in his/her development. The time of most rapid curve progression occurs during the time of greatest growth. A history and physical exam provides the clinician with an accurate picture of where the child is on his/her growth curve. Important factors to consider are the patient's sex, the Tanner stage, and the onset of menarche. In males, the onset of axillary hair correlates with menarche in females, although males will have approximately 24 months of growth left after the appearance of axillary hair. The importance of sex is evidenced by the equal number of males and females with small curves, but the predominance of females with larger curves. The Risser iliac apophysis ossification sign is an important radiographic measure of skeletal maturity (Table 43-1, Figure 43-1).

Table 43-1

Risser Sign

Risser 1	25% iliac apophysis ossification
Risser 2	50% iliac apophysis ossification
Risser 3	75% iliac apophysis ossification
Risser 4	100% ossification, with no fusion to iliac crest
Risser 5	Iliac apophysis fuses to iliac crest, indicating cessation of growth

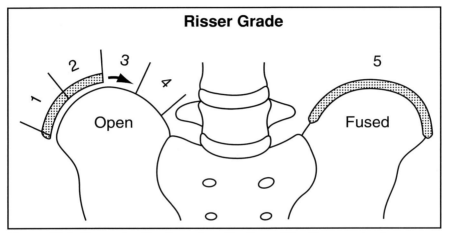

Figure 43-1. Risser classification of ossification of the iliac apophysis.

Curve progression is defined as an increase in Cobb angle of more than 5 degrees. In untreated patients with 20 to 30-degree curves, 68% of those with Risser grades 0 to 1 progressed, whereas only 23% of patients with Risser grades 2 to 4 had curve progression.[2] Therefore, the treatment of our case depends on the magnitude of the curve and where our 13-year-old girl is on her growth curve. Curves less than 20 degrees typically can be observed. For curves measuring 20 to 29 degrees, patients should be braced if they are Risser stage 0 to 1. In patients who are Risser stage 2 to 4, a progression of 5 degrees should be seen prior to bracing. Patients who present with curves measure 30 to 40 degrees should be braced immediately. For immature adolescents, surgery is indicated for thoracic curves of more than 40 degrees that progress despite bracing. Select thoracic curves greater than 30 degrees may require surgery if they are progressive and associated with thoracic lordosis. Select lumbar or thoracolumbar curves greater than 35 degrees associated with significant coronal imbalance and waist-line asymmetry may also be considered for surgery. In the mature adolescent patient, surgery is considered for curves greater than 50 degrees.

Another indication for surgery is if the deformity is unacceptable to the patient, usually because of cosmetic concerns or pain. It is rare that thoracic curves compromise pulmonary function, but this is occasionally seen in patients with large (>90 degree) curves or frank thoracic lordosis. If pulmonary compromise is present, then surgery is indicated.

In addition to these indications, sagittal deformity, rotation, and apical translation may contribute to unacceptable deformity and poor cosmesis. Sagittal deformities seen in scoliosis include thoracic lordosis, thoracic hyperkyphosis, thoracic hypokyphosis, thoracolumbar kyphosis, and lumbar kyphosis. These sagittal deformities can cause cervical pain, pulmonary dysfunction, and cosmetic problems. Rotational deformity may also result in an unsightly rib hump.

The indications for surgical correction of idiopathic adolescent scoliosis are based on the natural history of the disease and the predicted effects of the curve as the patient ages.[3] It is important to realize that these methods are based on population data and may not fit a particular patient. Additionally, the natural history of idiopathic adolescent scoliosis is not known with certainty and can be variable between patients. Therefore, surgical decision making should be done on a case-by-case basis for the best results using these indications as a guide.

References

1. Lonstein JE. Scoliosis: surgical vs non-surgical treatment. *Clin Orthop Relat Res.* 2006;443:248-259.
2. Lonstein JE, Carlson JM. The prediction of curve progression in untreated idiopathic scoliosis during growth. *J Bone Joint Surg Am.* 1984;66:1061-1071.
3. Bridwell KH. Surgical treatment of idiopathic adolescent scoliosis. *Spine.* 1999;24:2607-2616.

44

I HAVE A 64-YEAR-OLD FEMALE WHO IS SUFFERING FROM BACK PAIN AND NEUROGENIC CLAUDICATION SECONDARY TO FLATBACK SYNDROME. WHAT IS THE DIFFERENCE BETWEEN A SMITH-PETERSON AND PEDICLE SUBTRACTION OSTEOTOMY?

Yu-Po Lee, MD

Flatback syndrome was initially described in 1973 by Doherty after posterior spinal fusion for scoliosis, and the term was coined by Moe and Denis shortly after the original description. These initial reports described this complication of the Harrington rod system, which combines straight rods with distractive forces, leading to the obligatory loss of lumbar lordosis. Indeed, the most common cause of iatrogenic loss of lumbar lordosis or flatback syndrome is extension of distraction instrumentation into the lower lumbar spine.[1] In flatback syndrome, the rigid segment is compensated for by hyperextending the uninvolved cephalad segments and flexing the hips and knees.

Flatback after posterior lumbar fusion occurs from the failure to maintain or enhance lumbar lordosis and results in accelerated adjacent segment disease and loss of sagittal balance.[2] Sagittal balance is the relationship of the head and neck to the sacrum in standing position and can be measured by a plumb line from the body of C7 that should drop through the L5-S1 disc. In addition to a malaligned hypolordotic fusion, other common etiologies of flatback syndrome include pseudarthosis and breakdown of adjacent segments cephalad or caudad to the fusion mass. The flatback deformity results in back pain from the lordotic segment and from other areas of the spine that are compensating for the deformity.

Generally, conservative treatment of flatback syndrome yields poor results. Therefore, corrective surgery is frequently required, and a variety of osteotomies are available including the Smith-Peterson and pedicle subtraction osteotomies (Figures 44-1A and B). Corrective osteotomies are performed at the site of maximal deformity, although typically we perform them below L2 to minimize conus medullaris injury.

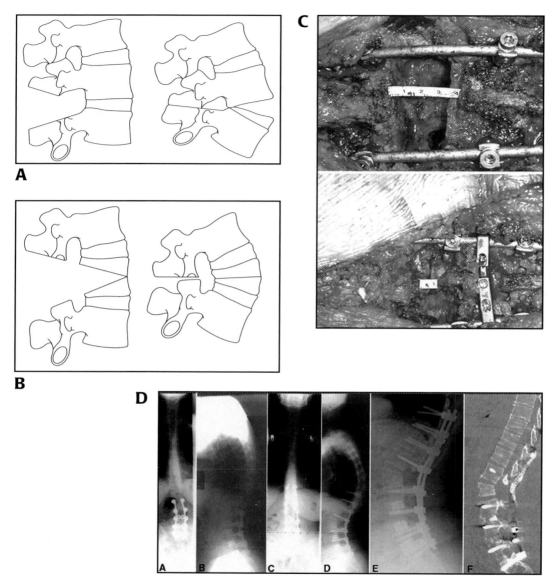

Figure 44-1. (A) Smith-Peterson osteotomy. Center of rotation is the posterior vertebral body (middle column). (B) Pedicle subtraction osteotomy. Center of rotation is the anterior vertebral body (anterior column). (C) Intraoperative photograph of a PSO demonstrating closure of the osteotomy site. (D) The first 2 images show preoperative radiographs of flat back syndrome after a lumbar fusion. The following 4 images are postoperative radiographs after an L2 PSO, showing restoration of lumbar lordosis.

The Smith-Peterson or extension osteotomy was described in 1945 and was the first posterior spinal osteotomy for correction of sagittal imbalance. Resection of the posterior elements and undercutting of the spinous processes is performed. Correction is achieved by posterior instrumentation in compression mode with the intervertebral disc opening anteriorly. A Smith-Peterson osteotomy results in approximately 1 degree of correction for each millimeter of posterior bone resected, and studies have shown that approximately 10 degrees of correction can be expected for a given procedure. In our experience, 3 or more segments are usually required to correct a typical flatback deformity.

The pedicle subtraction osteotomy is a 3-column posterior closing wedge osteotomy with the hinge on the anterior cortex.[3] At the desired level, all posterior elements including the pedicles and cephalad and caudal facet joints are removed. This allows access to the vertebral body where a posterior V-shaped wedge of bone is removed for deformity correction, leaving the anterior cortex intact. The osteotomy is closed using posterior instrumentation in compression mode. Because the pedicles are removed, the exiting nerve root shares a common foramen with the cephalad nerve root. When compression is applied, it is important to ensure that these neural elements are not damaged. The major advantages of the pedicle subtraction osteotomy over the Smith-Peterson osteotomy are the ability to reestablish lumbar lordosis with surgery at a single level and preserve length of the anterior column, reducing the risk of vascular injury. In patients with the flatback deformity, 26 to 34 degrees of correction have been obtained using this method.

In conclusion, the Smith-Peterson and pedicle subtraction osteotomies both restore lordosis in the flatback deformity after lumber fusion. The pedicle subtraction osteotomy is a more technically demanding surgery but has the advantages of restoring lumbar lordosis with surgery at a single level and a larger surface of cancellous bone apposition that theoretically decreases the risk of psuedarthrosis. Spine surgeons should be familiar with both of these techniques because they can be very effective in correcting sagittal alignment.[4] I typically use Smith-Peterson osteotomies if my deformity spans several levels and I want a gradual correction. If the deformity is very focal, then I would use a pedicle subtraction osteotomy. It is important to keep in mind that both methods are associated with a number of serious complications and significant blood loss (Figures 44-1C and D).

References

1. Potter BK, Lenke LG, Kuklo T. Prevention and management of iatrogenic flatback deformity. *J Bone Joint Surg-Am.* 2004;86:1793-1808.
2. Bridwell KH, Lenke LG, Lewis SJ. Treatment of spinal stenosis and fixed sagittal imbalance. *Clin Orthop Relat Res.* 2001;384:35-44.
3. Bridwell KH, Lewis SJ, Rinella A, et al. Pedicle subtraction osteotomy for the treatment of fixed sagittal imbalance: surgical technique. *J Bone Joint Surg-Am.* 2004;86:44-49.
4. Cho KJ, Bridwell KH, Lenke LG, et al. Comparison of Smith-Peterson versus pedicle subtraction osteotomy for correction of fixed sagittal imbalance. *Spine.* 2005;30:2030-2037.

45

I Have a 57-Year-Old Female Who Was Treated for Cervical Myelopathy 10 Years Ago With a Cervical Laminectomy. Her Myelopathy Is Getting Worse and She Is Unable to Extend Her Neck. Why Is Her Neurological Status Worsening?

Yu-Po Lee, MD

This woman is most likely having myelopathy secondary to postlaminectomy kyphosis. Cervical kyphosis is the most frequently seen cervical deformity, and the most common cause is iatrogenic secondary to an uninstrumented laminectomy. The cause of cervical kyphosis and its propensity for progression can best be understood by evaluating the biomechanics of cervical sagittal alignment.

Normal lordotic alignment of the cervical spine (C2 to C7) averages 14.4 degrees. The normal sagittal weight-bearing axis lies posterior to the vertebral bodies of C2 to C7. Cadavaric studies show that the posterior columns formed by the facet joints and articular processes support approximately 64% of the load seen in the neck. Because the posterior elements are responsible for most of the load transmission in the cervical spine, loss of integrity of the posterior bony and muscular architecture can cause instability and lead to a progressive kyphotic deformity. With a loss of normal sagittal cervical alignment, the weight-bearing axis shifts anteriorly. This loss of sagittal balance places the cervical musculature at a significant mechanical disadvantage and subsequently requires constant muscular contraction to maintain the head in an upright posture. Subsequently, fatigue and pain occur while the kyphosis progresses. The kyphotic progression causes most weight to be borne by the discs and anterior vertebral bodies. This increased pressure leads to progressive disc degeneration and further kyphosis. As the kyphosis progresses, the spinal cord becomes increasingly draped over the posterior aspect of the vertebral bodies.

Studies demonstrate that children have the highest incidence of postlaminectomy cervical kyphosis. Some believe that wedging of the anterior vertebral bodies is caused by compression of the cartilaginous endplates. Clinical studies in adults do not show a significant incidence of postlaminectomy kyphosis when there is normal preoperative alignment and no instability. However, any pre-existing kyphosis significantly increases the risk of forming postlaminectomy kyphosis after cervical laminectomy. The amount of facet resection is believed to correlate with the degree of instability after cervical laminectomy. Nowinski and colleagues reported that kyphosis was induced by as little as a 25% facetectomy in the presence of a laminectomy and suggested that prophylactic fusion be considered after performing a multilevel laminectomy.[1] Furthermore, detachment of the cervical extensor musculature from C2 is discouraged because it is believed to be a contributing factor in the initiation of cervical kyphosis.

The patient described here fits the natural history of someone who has postlaminectomy kyphosis. She did well initially but is now having myelopathy as her cord drapes over the kyphotic deformity. After a thorough history and physical examination, appropriate imaging studies are necessary. Plain radiographs including flexion-extension views are helpful to determine the degree of the kyphosis as well as the flexibility of the kyphosis. Ankylosis must be ruled out, because its presence might necessitate an osteotomy to correct the defomity.[2] A CT scan is helpful in determining the presence of ankylosis. Also, it is useful in visualizing the vertebral arteries. Magnetic resonance imagery (MRI) is also helpful in evaluating cord changes, including myelomalacia, syrinx formation, and cord atrophy.

References

1. Nowinski GP, Visarious H, Nolte LP, Herkowitz HN. A biomechanical comparison of cervical laminoplasty and cervical laminectomy with progressive facetectomy. *Spine.* 1993;18:1995-2004.
2. Albert TJ, Vacarro A. Postlaminectomy kyphosis. *Spine.* 1998;23(24):2738-2745.

46

I HAVE A 62-YEAR-OLD FEMALE WITH RHEUMATOID ARTHRITIS WHO HAS NOW BECOME MYELOPATHIC. DOES SHE NEED AN OPERATION?

Yu-Po Lee, MD

Rheumatoid arthritis (RA) is a chronic, systemic autoimmune disorder. The destructive synovitis seen in rheumatoid arthritis is believed to be the result of an autoimmune response to an antigen expressed by the synovial cells. Spinal disease eventually occurs in about 60% of patients with RA. Patients with more severe and longer duration of disease are at higher risk for cervical spine involvement. Once instability begins, the disease tends to progress to more complex instability patterns. In particular, atlantoaxial subluxation tends to progress toward superior migration of the odontoid. Rheumatoid synovitis may affect the synovial joints around the dens. This leads to erosion of the dens and progressive damage of the transverse, alar, and apical ligaments, leading to atlantoaxial subluxation. Pannus formation posterior to the dens may further contribute to cord compression. Superior migration of the odontoid occurs from bony erosion between the occipitoatlantal and atlantoaxial joints or bilateral erosion of the lateral masses. This can result in brainstem compression and vascular compromise to the basivertebral and anterior spinal arteries. Erosion of the facet joints and degeneration of the interspinous ligaments may lead to subluxation of the subaxial spine. Multiple-level subluxations may lead to a "stepladder" appearance or a kyphotic deformity (Figures 46-1 and 46-2).

The clinical presentation of RA is variable and ranges from asymptomatic patients to those with severe deformity and neurologic compromise. The Ranawat classification is often used for myelopathy classification (Table 46-1).

Lateral radiographs are the most helpful for initial evaluation of the cervical spine. The posterior atlanto-dens interval (PADI), anterior atlanto-dens interval (ADI), subaxial sub-

Figure 46-1. Sagittal MRI demonstrating a retro-odontoid pannus with upper cervical spinal cord compression.

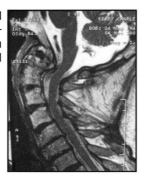

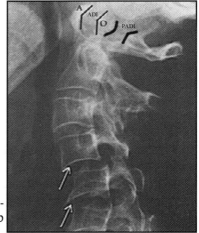

Figure 46-2. Lateral cervical radiograph demonstrating atlantoaxial instability (C1-2) and stair-step spondylolisthesis at C4-5 and C5-6.

Table 46-1
Ranawat Classification of Rheumatoid Arthritis[3]

Class	Definition
I	Patients have no neurologic deficit.
II	Patients have subjective weakness, dysesthesias, and hyperreflexia.
III	Patients have objective signs of weakness and upper motor signs.
IIIA	Patients are ambulatory.
IIIB	Patients are not ambulatory.

luxation, and superior migration of the odontoid should be evaluated. Flexion-extension lateral cervical radiographs are useful for evaluation of dynamic instability. An anterior ADI greater than 3.5 mm is considered abnormal. However, the posterior ADI has more prognostic value.[1] An anterior ADI greater than 9 to 10 mm and posterior ADI less than 14 mm are associated with an increased risk of neurologic injury and usually require surgery. Diagnosing superior migration of the odontoid can be difficult. Further evalution with magenetic resonance imaging (MRI) or CT is recommended.

Treatment of RA is based on medical and surgical management to alleviate pain and prevent neurologic injury. Surgery is considered for patients with intractable pain or neurologic deficits. Surgical intervention should be attempted before the onset of Ranawat class III myelopathy because neurologic improvement is limited after presentation. C1-C2 fusion is recommended for patients with a posterior ADI less than 14 mm or if there is more than 3.5 mm of segmental mobility.[2,3] Fusion may be performed with wires, transarticular C1-C2 screws, or C1 lateral mass screws with C2 isthmic, pedicle, or laminar screws. If basilar invagination has occurred, an occiput to C2 fusion is recommended.

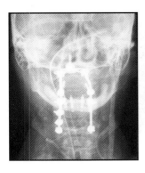 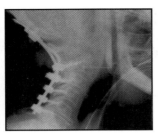

Figure 46-3. Postoperative AP/lateral radiographs that demonstrate a C1-2 laminectomy and an occipital-cervical fusion (occiput-C6).

Decompression may be accomplished with a C1 arch removal or transoral odontoid resection (Figure 46-3).

References

1. Boden SD, Dodge LD, Bohlman HH, et al. Rheumatoid arthritis of the cervical spine: a long-term analysis with predictors of paralysis and recovery. *J Bone Joint Surg Am.* 1993;75(9):1282-1297.
2. Clark CR, Goetz DD, Menezes AH. Arthrodesis of the cervical spine in rheumatoid arthritis. *J Bone Joint Surg Am.* 1989;71(3):381-392.
3. Ranawat CS, O'Leary P, Pellicci P, et al. Cervical spine fusion in rheumatoid arthritis. *J Bone Joint Surg Am.* 1979;61(7):1003-1010.

SECTION XV

REHABILITATION

I Have a Patient With Discogenic Pain and Was Going to Prescribe Him Physical Therapy. What Is the Difference Between Williams and McKenzie Exercises?

Joseph D. Smucker, MD

Williams flexion exercises, described by Dr. Paul Williams, were published in a 1937 text.[1] Such exercises were developed to moderate the balance between paraspinal/extensor groups of the lumbar spine and abdominal or flexor groups in this same region.[2] These exercises hope to provide an overall increase in trunk stability in the lumbar region by actively developing "core" muscle groups in the abdomen, posterior hip musculature, and posterior thighs.

Since their original description, these exercises have been used for the nonoperative management of a number of low back conditions including those associated with spinal stenosis. Examples of such exercises include pelvic tilt, knee to the chest, double knee to the chest, partial sit-ups, hamstring and hip flexor stretching, and squat exercises. This regimen is often performed under the direction of a physical therapist and may be easily prescribed as "Williams-type" exercises.[3]

In contrast to Williams exercises, the McKenzie approach focuses on the restoration of lumbar lordosis via an extension-based treatment of acute low back pain.[4] Postural dysfunction, such as the lack of normal lumbar lordosis, is theorized to result in migration of the intervertebral disc into pain-sensitive structures. McKenzie exercises are often used in patients with discogenic pain because it avoids positioning in flexion that often exacerbates patient's symptoms.

Once the patient is given a mechanical diagnosis and has been specifically classified, they are then treated with a combination of postural adjustments, exercises specific to their condition, and occasionally spinal mobilization or manipulation. McKenzie methods also focus on identifying a directional preference; that is, patients who have back pain with certain patterns of movement are told to avoid motions that increase back pain and move into positions that are more comfortable.[4] Terms such as directional preference, centralization, and peripheralization have been used as condition descriptors.[5]

References

1. Williams P. Lesions of the lumbosacral spine: chronic traumatic (postural) destruction of the intervertebral disc. *Bone Joint Surg.* 1937;29:690-703.
2. Nachemson A. The influence of spinal movements on the lumbar intradiscal pressure and on the tensile stresses in the annulus fibrosis. *Acta Orthop Scand.* 1963;33:183-207.
3. Williams P. *The Lumbosacral Spine.* New York: McGraw Hill; 1965:80-98.
4. Ponte D, Jensen G, Kent B. A preliminary report on the use of McKenzie protocol versus Williams protocol in the treatment of low back pain. *J Orthop Sports Phys Ther.* 1984;6:130-139.
5. Machado LA, de Souza MS, Ferreira PH, et al. The McKenzie method for low back pain: a systematic review of the literature with a meta-analysis approach. *Spine.* 2006;31:E254-E262.

I ALWAYS TELL MY PATIENTS THAT THE MAJORITY OF DISC HERNIATIONS AND RADICULOPATHY GET BETTER WITH TIME. ARE THERE ANY NONOPERATIVE MODALITIES I CAN PROVIDE THEM WITH IN THE INTERIM?

Joseph D. Smucker, MD

Spine surgeons are often involved in the nonoperative management of patients with lumbar disc herniations. Many patients who enter a surgical practice automatically assume that their condition will be best treated with a surgical procedure. Although this is certainly not the intent of the referring physician, moderating the thought process in the patient-physician relationship is sometimes challenging. A large component in the management of disc herniations and radiculopathy is one of patient education.

The educational process begins with drawings and models of the lumbar spine, describing to the patient the function and potential dysfunction of the intervertebral discs. Personally, I like to initiate several nonoperative modalities in patients with disc herniations and radiculopathy. Oral corticosteroids are an effective medication for mitigating acute radicular symptoms. A medrol (IVEX Pharmaceutical, Miami, FL) dose pack can help the patient rapidly resolve an acute radicular episode. I also start the patient on a nonsteroidal, anti-inflammatory drug (NSAID), which will help to reduce the inflammatory response associated with a herniated nucleus pulposus.

Low dose, short-term narcotic pain medications can be effective in moderating the symptoms of radiculopathy. Long-term opioid use has no role in the treatment of disc herniations and will only lead to increased pain sensitivity and narcotic addiction. I often advise my patients to observe a strict weight-lifting restriction during the first 6 weeks of their treatment. It is my preference to minimize lifting to no more than 5 to 10 pounds during this period and to also minimize bending and twisting. These activity modifications theoretically reduce the stress imparted to the damaged intervertebral disc.[1,2]

Physical therapy is an essential part of the early and intermediate treatment of those patients with disc herniations. Initially, modalities may be helpful such as electrical stimulation and massage therapy to help reduce paraspinal muscle spasm. Stretching and range of motion help provide flexibility to patients who are deconditioned from immobilization. Patients are then taught proper ergonomics and body positioning to minimize chances of a similar episode occurring.

As mentioned previously, these simple steps—including patient education, oral corticosteroids, NSAIDs, and physical therapy—can effectively manage more than 90% of lumbar disc herniations. For those patients with persistent symptoms, epidural steroid injections and surgical intervention may be warranted.[3,4]

References

1. Weinstein JN, Tosteson TD, Lurie JD, et al. Surgical vs nonoperative treatment for lumbar disk herniation: the Spine Patient Outcomes Research Trial (SPORT), a randomized trial. *JAMA*. 2006;296:2441-2450.
2. Atlas SJ, Keller RB, Wu YA, et al. Long-term outcomes of surgical and nonsurgical management of sciatica secondary to a lumbar disc herniation: 10 year results from the Maine lumbar spine study. *Spine*. 2005;30:927-935.
3. Loupasis GA, Stamos K, Katonis PG, et al. Seven- to 20-year outcome of lumbar discectomy. *Spine*. 1999;24:2313-2317.
4. Osterman H, Seitsalo S, Karppinen J, et al. Effectiveness of microdiscectomy for lumbar disc herniation: a randomized controlled trial with 2 years of follow-up. *Spine*. 2006;31:2409-2414.

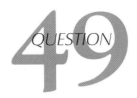

I Have a Patient With a Complete Spinal Cord Injury Who Was Treated With a Posterior Thoracolumbar Fusion. What Are the Postoperative Medical Complications Associated With Patients Who Have This Type of Injury?

Joseph D. Smucker, MD

In my clinical practice, the surgical management of spinal cord injury as a result of trauma is relatively common. This patient population is predominately young and male, although occasionally those with long-standing cervical or other spinal stenoses have similar injuries as a result of minor trauma such as a fall.

It is my personal preference to initiate an early, multidisciplinary approach to the management of these patients. Even prior to surgery, common challenges such as neurogenic spinal shock may be overlooked. Timing of surgical intervention in patients with spinal cord injury has been very controversial.[1] It is my preference to take patients to surgery to stabilize and/or treat their spinal cord injuries as soon as medically appropriate. I believe this helps to reduce potential medical complications that may arise from prolonged immobilization of patients with unstable spinal injuries.

Common postoperative medical complications include pulmonary injuries as simple as atelectasis and as devastating as adult respiratory distress syndrome.[2,3] Urological dysfunction is also associated with spinal cord injury and may result in infection. Patients are taught at a very early stage the importance of self-catherization.

Throughout the hospital and postoperative course, it is important to maintain appropriate deep venous thrombosis (DVT) prophylaxis.[4] DVT prophylaxis at a minimum should include thromboembolic deterrent (TED) hose stockings and lower-extremity, mechanical compression devices. Patients should also be started on anticoagulants such as aspirin, warfarin, or enoxaparin. On several occasions, I have placed an inferior vena caval filter for those patients at high risk for bleeding-associated complications or for those patients who have demonstrated DVT on a screening ultrasound study.

A patient with an injured spinal cord also has significant challenges in the immediate and intermediate period with regard to mobilization. As the result of sensory deficits from a spinal cord injury, patients are at an increased risk for wound complications associated with pressure ulcers. Again, appropriate teaching of patient and family members is critical to avoid such issues even in the long term.

Autonomic dysreflexia manifests as an abnormal physiologic response to common medical diagnoses such as constipation, urinary tract infections, or skin ulcers. This condition can be deadly to patients with spinal cord injury if unrecognized, and may manifest as severe hypertension.[5] Appropriate teaching and monitoring is the key to successful long-term outcomes with this condition.

Lastly, patients with spinal cord injuries suffer from a variety of psychosocial issues. It is important to not underestimate the devastating effect the loss of independence may have on an individual. Familial, religious, and psychiatric support is essential in preventing these patients from suffering life-threatening depression. Patients should be watched closely for early signs of depression, and social support services and medications should be instituted early.

References

1. Fehlings MG, Perrin RG. The timing of surgical intervention in the treatment of spinal cord injury: a systematic review of recent clinical evidence. *Spine.* 2006;31:S28-S35.
2. McKinley W, McNamee S, Meade M, et al. Incidence, etiology, and risk factors for fever following acute spinal cord injury. *J Spinal Cord Med.* 2006;29:501-506.
3. McKinley W, Meade MA, Kirshblum S, et al. Outcomes of early surgical management versus late or no surgical intervention after acute spinal cord injury. *Arch Phys Med Rehabil.* 2004;85:1818-1825.
4. Winemiller MH, Stolp-Smith KA, Silverstein MD, et al. Prevention of venous thromboembolism in patients with spinal cord injury: effects of sequential pneumatic compression and heparin. *J Spinal Cord Med.* 1999;22:182-191.
5. Karlsson AK. Autonomic dysfunction in spinal cord injury: clinical presentation of symptoms and signs. *Prog Brain Res.* 2006;152:1-8.

INDEX